HEART WARRIOR

In loving memory of my parents,
Adrian Allen and Lera Adella (Brown) Morgan

Contents

Prologue

Sitting on a cold, wooden bench in Budapest, Hungary, I could not wrap my mind around the information I had just received from Dr. Mározsán Ibolya. She had just told me that I had a torn aorta and needed immediate open-heart surgery, an aortic dissection. The Hungarian cardiologist had led me to that bench in the hallway of the Cardiology Hospital and told me to sit there while she went to prepare for this emergency surgery.

Surgery? Where, in Budapest? At the foot of the Buda Hills where I was living and had lived for 3 years? Have the surgery here? Statistics show 18% of those who suffer an aortic dissection die before arriving at the hospital; 21% die within 24 hours if they don't have surgery. Those are US statistics. How much worse could it be in a post-communist country just eight years after the change in government and western unification? I was not prepared for this news. I had not awakened that morning to grapple with such a decision!

My brain went into a deep fog; I longed for a safe place to clear my head. As a child I had escaped my father's anger by mental hiding places, sometimes by a stream with only the sounds of the water next to a meadow with horses peacefully grazing in the grass. Not this cold bench. I wanted to be somewhere that would help me think straight, like a mountain lake cabin with a roaring fire on a winter's evening. That place.

But, instead, I sat on a cold, hard, soviet style wooden bench far from the safety of home, family and friends. As I sat dazed and trying to clear my head, two nurses walked by me in the hallway and the smell of nicotine and lingering smoke hit me hard. What was it that Ibolya had just said—she was going to prepare to call in doctors and medical staff for surgery? Panic shot through my shock, and I knew I had to get out of there. I do not remember the steps to the front door. My next memory is walking into Város-major Park, a couple of streets away. I sat down on a bench there in hopes of clearing my head, but I can't sit, I must keep moving. I wasn't sure if my next moments could be, would be my last. I had to keep moving.

I had heard all of my life that when someone is facing death that their life flashes before their eyes. For the next 5 hours on that fateful Monday I roamed through the streets of Budapest with scenes and memories of my life flashing before me. I had walked away from the surgery that was to repair the dissection. I did the unthinkable with a time bomb in my chest. Maybe it was stupid, crazy, certainly a risky idea, but I had to do something. I had to try to get home to Nashville. I would soon go to Ferihegy Airport with the hope of flying to the States.

Killin' Snakes

My father had a great inquisitive mind and could build or repair anything electrical, plumbing, even light construction, but those talents had eluded me from the beginning. Both of my brothers, older and younger, inherited his amazing trait and talents that I wish I had. Because if my father could do it, and my brothers could do it, then Randall can do it. But I had no aptitude nor desire; therefore, in his eyes, I must be lazy and unwilling to learn. In his more patient moments, he would decide that he would once again try to teach me and, after a few tries of me hacking my way through, he would say, "You could do this, or that, if you didn't go at everything like you were killin' snakes."

I still think about that today when I am forced to do some basic repairs around the house that are simple for most people. But for me, yep, I still go at most things of this nature—*like I am killin' snakes.*

My father was a self-employed electrician who owned and operated Morgan Electric Company. I remember hearing more than once that his desire was to change that name to Morgan & Sons Electric in the years to come as we, his three sons, came of age and finished school. Unfortunately, I was the artistic kid with no abilities for electrical or anything having to do with 'fixing' things. When I picked up a screwdriver or a hammer there was always a good possibility that I would make a situation worse, or even destroy whatever it was that my father thought I could and should learn to fix.

Every Saturday morning, my father would announce the chores for the day. My older brother would always go with him to the garage or to some task that was repairing or making a plan to repair. My younger brother was four years younger than I, and he would play until he got old enough to join the Saturday workforce. Until my older brother left home—soon after high school graduation—I would be assigned to helping my mother in the house. Though I don't remember being overly thrilled at helping with interior house projects, I did want to help my mother because I loved her and felt safer with her than with my father. But it wasn't always housework for me, as I did work with my father on the bigger projects. When I did have to work with him, I usually ended up not paying attention or simply goofing off and that would make him angry. I did like painting, maybe because I enjoyed color and I could see immediate change with a paint brush that I certainly did not see when trying to thread a plumbing pipe or something equally as mundane. We had a brick home, and it seemed that we painted the trim and window shutters every few years. One year, we even reroofed the house, and though I enjoyed some aspects of being on the roof, it was hard work carrying all those bundles of shingles up that Morgan Electric Company extension ladder, which I still have in my basement to this day.

By my teen years, I had heard the phrase *you will never amount to anything* hundreds of times from my father. I was worthless to my father, whereas my older brother could take things apart just to see how they worked and put them back together with complete success. But my relationship with my father was not easy, largely due to my inabilities, or laziness in his eyes. When I was 17 and just out of high school, I purchased a 1965 Mustang convertible, dark blue with a white top and white roll and pleated interior, from

Joe Corley Motors on Gallatin Road, in East Nashville. It was the prettiest car I'd ever seen. One Saturday morning while eating breakfast, my father decided he wanted to teach me some basics in car care, specifically the engine on the Mustang. I remember the feeling of dread taking over my brain as I chewed my breakfast cereal. Even at 17 I realized there was no way out of a morning in the garage with my father *as long as you live under my roof* and all of that. He told me to get a wrench and loosen this and that and pretty soon the carburetor was off. Okay, nothing disastrous. After a lengthy explanation of the purpose of the carburetor, which traveled through one ear and out the other, he wanted me to put it back on the engine. Not being quite as stupid as he thought, I replaced the piece back where I had taken it off and began to tighten the screws. I just remember tightening it and him saying, "Give it one more good turn to make it snug," which I did with a bit more strength than needed, and it cracked the carburetor. Cracked! A perfectly good carburetor was ruined, and he went into a rage and that ended the well-intentioned mechanic lesson with both of us storming off. Yep, killin' snakes!

I was most likely a mirror that he did not find attractive. Having a similar sense of humor and an inherited quick wit landed me in more hot water than I CARE to remember. My father would sometimes say the same statement repeatedly, expressing his frustration with us, his family. Those repetitive statements would stick in my mind, and as I grew into my teen years, I found it almost impossible not to quip back with some of those statements. An example of that would be when he wanted to manipulate his family into submission over a disagreement he would say, "Why can't we be like other people?" That is harmless enough, but when I wanted to join my friends from our church youth group for an evening out, he would say no, and I would keep pushing and saying, "But other people are going." He would respond with, "Well, we are not like other people." So at a later time, when he would say, "Why can't we be like other people," I would quickly quip, "Because we are not like other people." That always ended badly. Thankfully, I was little and could run like the wind. And that's what I wanted to do that day in Budapest. I wanted to run like the wind, but I didn't have anywhere to go. I couldn't run from myself. So what I did next that day in Budapest was almost like killin' snakes.

Going Under the Third Time

The tear in my aorta happened while I was out with friends for a Sunday afternoon proverbial *three-hour tour* on a lake in Holland aboard a cabin cruiser. My friends, David and Evelyne (Oprel) Lloyd, had been working with me in Eastern Europe for a couple of years by this point. We sang together in one of our *Tramps* street bands. We had been in a number of countries in outreaches from Holland to Bulgaria, Turkey to Hungary, but with a real focus on Croatia and Sarajevo, after the tragic siege of the city from 1992-1996. The siege of Sarajevo—the capital of Bosnia and Herzegovina—was the longest siege of a capital city in the history of modern warfare. Ten thousand dead by some estimates—a toll so large that makeshift cemeteries had to be constructed all over the city. One such cemetery can be found in the middle of the 1984 Olympic arena, crumbling tombstones marking the graves of countless men, women and children killed by the violent conflict. Dave, Ev and I sang on the streets of Sarajevo as *buskers*-with purpose… to meet and minister to the hurting people that we met.

Dave and Ev had moved from Budapest and had been living in Zagreb, Croatia for a few months when they learned of their first pregnancy. Ev wanted to have the baby in the Netherlands so I drove down from Budapest and we packed them up and moved a large van full of furniture and all of their belongings from Croatia to Ev's parent's house in Delft. After a couple of days traveling, followed by unloading and moving all their items up the narrow

Dutch stairs into the 3rd floor rooms, we were exhausted. Her parents, always hospitable, had borrowed a friend's boat for the next day, a Sunday afternoon restful day in the sun, or so we thought.

Dave and Ev had ventured out paddling in a small dingy a little way from the main boat, when I decided to swim out to them and share a few laughs before returning to the main boat for a nap. As I swam back, I went to the far side of the boat where I was no longer in view of the dingy, when a sharp pain paralyzed me. When I say sharp pain—think of the possibility of a cannonball going through your chest and exiting your back, because that is what it felt like to me. The pain immediately paralyzed me in the water. I was unable to take a breath or move my limbs. I remember going under the first time and feeling relieved to resurface before going down a second time. At this point, my mind realized I was most likely going to drown. When I went down the third time, my memory said *You don't come back up from the third time down.* Horror! Remember, at this point, I am unable to move my arms and legs. I gasped for air, not able to speak and certainly not able to yell for help. I was behind the boat, so no one could see I was in danger. I just kept saying the name of Jesus, over and over in my mind. When I popped up from the third time down, I was able to gasp another small amount of air into my lungs. During these seconds, which felt like an eternity, my body had floated toward the boat. There was a little lip of molding just at the waterline on that large cabin cruiser, so I did my best to get an inch of my shoulder to hang on. Anything to stay afloat. As I bobbed up-and-down, but miraculously staying above water, my body continued to move along the side of the boat until finally reaching the back where there was a ladder. I was so relieved to float up against the ladder, and in time I gained enough feeling to get my hand to take hold. I was able to rest a little longer with a hold on the ladder, and little-by-little the feeling in my limbs returned. Finally, I was able to climb into the boat. I remember walking to the table where Ada, Ev's mom sat reading a magazine, and I sat down in the chair next to her, and she began telling me about this article that she was reading. I could hear her words but was unable to form words of my own at that point, so I sat there in silence. In a few minutes—time was still moving very slowly as if I were in some sort of time warp—I decided I needed to lie down so I got up and moved to a bunk underneath the front deck. I was resting there but was afraid and asking God, in my silent prayers, for his wisdom and guidance in what to do next.

Eventually, I heard my friends return to the boat from their dingy excursion. They climbed aboard and started talking with her mom and after some time I heard David ask where I was. Soon he came looking and found me on the bunk and asked if I was alright. I was able to say simply *no, my heart*, or something along those lines. I did finally convince him this was not a joke. I was in trouble and needed medical help. With all best intentions, Ev brought me a glass of sherry to thin my blood, as we thought I must have had a heart attack. So I sipped on the sherry, which was delicious I might add, as they pulled anchor and set out for the shore.

It seemed forever to get the boat docked and everything put away and secured. I have wondered since why we did not call for an ambulance, but I think I was the only one who really understood the severity of what I was feeling. I guess, the longer it took to get to the hospital the more time I had to convince myself that I was fine. Nothing serious. By the time we left the boat, drove in the car back to Delft, it had to be three, or more hours before I was at the Emergency Room.

At the ER, once again there wasn't any real sense of urgency as I waited in a chair in the waiting room. Finally taken back and placed on a gurney, I gave my account of the incident to a young woman, whom I believe was in her residency. After a short examination with her stethoscope she pronounced that everything seemed fine. She then hooked me up to an electrocardiogram machine and found that my heart was functioning well. She wanted me to have a stress test and explained to me that would be on a bicycle. Unfortunately, it was late evening on Sunday, and it would need to wait until tomorrow.

In Holland, the land of bicycle travel, one should know that a bicycle would be the ultimate test. I entertained myself with such thoughts as I lay on the gurney wondering, hoping.

She thought it best for me to be observed overnight in cardiac intensive care. Someone came and took me farther into the hospital and placed me in a small room, a ward with three other men. Though I had lived briefly in the Netherlands and was used to Dutch culture, I was still surprised when they brought the coffee cart around that evening for a *coffee* while hooked up to heart monitoring machines. Seriously, a cup of coffee before bed in intensive cardiac care? Hey, when in Rome, and I had a delicious cup of caffeine which probably did not help with what happened next.

I had a panic attack! I had heard of panic attacks a number of times in my life, but I had no real idea of what they might feel like. I was lying in bed trying to quiet my mind so that I could hopefully get some sleep between the breathing, snores and beeps of the multiple machines monitoring us four men in this room that was not any larger than a normal bedroom. At first, my body went hot, not warm, but red hot with immediate perspiration popping out of every pore. My heart started pounding so strongly and loudly that I was sure the other men in the room could hear it. My heart pounded in my ears, and I remember the thought, the desire, the fear of pulling my IV out and running. It didn't matter where. I just had to get out of there. I had to get outside and run!

I called for the nurse who came at a fast clip. She knew by looking at me that I was in distress. She immediately started patting my arm and locked eyes with mine.

She said, "You are okay . You are just reacting to the medicine. You are going to be fine."

She had a kind and gentle tone. Much softer than her previous tones with the men in her charge.

That was my first panic attack. When people tell me today, they suffer with panic attacks, I no longer downplay it in my mind, thinking they are just being dramatic and are feeling a bit anxious. My heart goes out to them. I completely understand and empathize.

My second panic attack was not far behind the first, as I awoke sometime predawn to find another team of nurses removing the IV from the man in the bed immediately in front of me. We were toe-to-toe with a small walk space between us. I had talked with him briefly the night before, even though he was struggling to breathe. Now I awoke to find him no longer alive. The nurses were quietly trying to get him unhooked and removed from the room. I watched with sadness, but also fear, and the panic attack hit. My body flushed with heat and my heart pounded stronger than before. I could not catch my breath. I would be following this man in death at any moment. One of the nurses removing the man across from me heard my gasps for air and walked over and comforted me. She also recognized what was going on and I think she had been made aware by the nurse of the previous evening that I had already experienced some degree of panic.

The man's death did not help my mental state, as I tried to remain hopeful and continue in prayer for God's healing. I was constantly praying—without ceasing as it were.

Monday morning I was told that they were taking me down for the treadmill test. After a restless night and the early morning trauma of death, I was not feeling very safe and secure, wondering if I would die! The stress test could kill me. On the stationary bike, they had me wired for sound by those little electrodes glued to my chest and then told me to pedal. As I pedaled, trying hard to obey, I began to burn in that very place in my back where I had felt the cannonball exit the day before. When I turned to tell the supervisor of the test, he was holding his head in his hands and not even looking at the heart monitor. I asked him somewhat breathlessly if he was okay, and he said he had just had his wisdom teeth out. What? Wait, seriously? I immediately stopped pedaling—despite his protests—and climbed off the bicycle. I had them take me back to my room, and I called David to come and collect me. At that time, I had no idea the risk I was taking. I just wanted to go home, home to Budapest.

— 3 —

Della

I was raised in the Nashville suburb of Inglewood just east of downtown Nashville. In the 1950's, Nashville had one skyscraper, with 30 floors—the L&C Tower. In 2022, the skyline boasts a number of high-rise buildings making it hard to even find the L&C. That 30 floor tower was the home of the Life and Casualty Insurance Company, which was instrumental in the development of the world-renown, oldest radio show, The Grand Ole Opry.

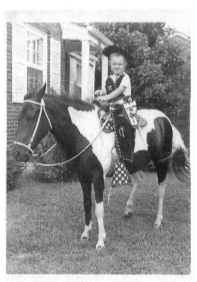

Inglewood was a 10-minute drive from downtown and was largely a 1940-50s ranch-style neighborhood with quiet tree lined streets. There was a feeling of being known in the community where you attended school, church and most activities. Seemed like every year of my early years a man came around in the summer with his pony and would take your picture mounted on the pony.

In our community children could ride their bikes safely for hours. My bike was a metallic-gold three-speed Western Flyer from Western Auto on Gallatin Road near East High School. My parents gave me the bike for Christmas and I practically lived on my bicycle through my elementary and high school years.

When I started junior high school, I was younger in age and in development than most of the kids in the 7th grade. Some of the boys appeared to be already through puberty and looked adult compared to me. I was short, skinny, auburn-headed, and insecure. I wished I could go back to elementary school where I felt comfortable. My elementary school was small, and this new world of junior high school was a magnet for a number of schools in the area.

Nashville was still relatively small and safe back then. I was a teenager before we locked our doors at night. I remember that because I was a sleepwalker, and early one morning the milk man—who delivered milk in glass bottles in a truck full of large chunks of smooth ice—knocked on the kitchen door, waking my parents to say, "Mr. Morgan, your son is on your front porch." Sure enough, sometime in the night I had wandered from my bed and curled up to finish my night's sleep on the front porch. This might be the reason my parents started locking the doors.

My mother, Adella or Della, as her sisters called her, was the middle daughter of seven girls. Even though she struggled with her self-esteem, she was smart and determined. When I married in 1975, my mother gave me her well-worn high school ring from Burns High School, Burns, Tennessee Class of 1941. I wore it on special occasions as a pinky ring—we wore too much jewelry in the 70s, with our gold choker chains and rings. When the gold medallion culture changed, I put her ring in a lockbox where it remained for many years. When I was ordained a pastor in 2014, I wore the ring to the service and have worn it every day since. My mother had always prayed for me, and I wanted to honor her by having something of hers with me every day.

I remember once when my mother told one of my aunts, my father's youngest sister, that she believed that I would preach in churches one day. Well, my aunt and I both had a good laugh over that. But mothers know things; she believed in God and His amazing power, and she knew my heart better than I, even despite my mouth and seeming lack of a filter.

My mother used to say, "Randall, you don't have to say everything you think."

I would respond, "I don't."

That resulted in a bewildered expression on her face, as if to say, "Oh no, what is he not saying?"

My mother had a good sense of humor, which I am not sure most people realized. I saw it and loved it. Nothing made me happier than to make her smile and laugh. Often, she would press her index finger to her lips when I was being cheeky (borrowing a British term), which was often. But I thought she was just composing herself and measuring her response. But it occurred to me one day that she was actually suppressing a smile or a laugh. It was a lightbulb moment. All those years I had made her smile and wasn't aware of it!

Probably because I had such a difficult relationship with my father, with no closeness or affection, my mother was my rock. She was the stability in our home on an emotional level. My father provided for us and he worked hard, but he was absent emotionally.

The worst memory of my childhood was autumn of 1966 when I was in the first months of my 7th grade year at Isaac Litton Junior High School. I was already feeling insecure and vulnerable in my school class, and to add to the trauma of that season, my mother had a large growth that developed under her jawline that seemed to get bigger by the day. Before Christmas of that year was the first time I can remember hearing the word *cancer* being whispered. Just after Christmas, she had surgery and afterwards was diagnosed with Hodgkin's disease. I was told that she wouldn't live long with Hodgkin's, so I lived day and night believing she might die at any time.

Living under this pressure added to my already insecure feelings, being in a larger school with much larger or more mature children. That school year was so hard that it is just a blur of sadness and dark shadows in my mind.

In the years that would follow, my mother's cancer caused reoccurring tumors. Almost yearly, new malignancies would surface, and she would undergo radiation treatments. Only the first one required surgery. But it seemed every Christmas might be her last. My father would actually say every season leading up to Christmas, "This will probably be your mother's last Christmas." This would horrify me and shake me to the core. I could not imagine life without my mother. She was my rock. I know my father loved her and was afraid of losing her, but sometime I think he used her sickness to try and control my behavior, but it was cruel and made Christmas a hard season for me. On one hand my most favorite time of the year, but on the other hand it was the hardest and saddest time as well. It is truly the most wonderful time of the year, and yet it can bring up sudden sadness and pain even now.

My fear of losing my mother was so strong and constant in my teen years. I used to have nightmares in which she was in trouble but I was unable to help her. I can still remember two of those dreams to this day. One was a car accident at the end of our driveway, where the car just spun into a pile of metal with her inside. But I could not free her. I tried, while everyone else just stood there watching, unable or unwilling to help. Then the car would burst into flames and I would awaken in a sweat. In the other nightmare we would be at church. I'd watch her leave the pew beside my father and go the ladies room, and I knew she was going in there to die. But I could not go in, and, once again, I could not get anyone to help. Both were recurring and so horribly vivid. Those nightmares felt so real, but I didn't have anyone in which to share those fears. The closest person in my life was my mother and I would never talk of death with her because I was not brave enough to face that conversation.

I valued my time with her, so I did not mind being assigned tasks in the house. She told me stories of her childhood growing up on the banks of the Harpeth River. She taught me manners, and how to behave socially, and in other's homes. We would often sing while working around the house and I learned vocal parts from her beautiful alto voice. As a first tenor, I am still attracted to the alto part. Those who have sung with me on worship teams can attest to this.

She was the middle of seven girls on the Brown side, and my father was the eldest boy of nine children on the Morgan side. I had 28 aunts and uncles, 4 grandparents, and they all loved Della. She was kind and compassionate to everyone, which contributed to her being the sweetheart of both sides of the family. I remember that both sides of the family came to pray when she was in the hospital having that first tumor removed. But even as a young teen I noticed that despite their prayers and confidence in their faith, they never seemed to give God the credit for her healing, her 17-year extension of life. The family, instead of saying that God had healed her, would say things like, "W*ell, doctors just don't know, do they?*" or to her in a jovial moment, "*Adella, they will have to hit you on the head on Judgment Day.*" Southerners have colorful expressions, which I love, but I may have been confused by the lack of credit given to God.

Despite the early diagnosis and negative prognosis, my mother lived 17 years with Hodgkin's disease. She crossed over in 1980 just a couple of weeks after her 57th birthday, losing her battle with breast cancer. I think her body was just not strong enough to fight the chemo after so many years of radiation treatments from the Hodgkin's malignancies. She was a fighter and had very strong faith in her God. She told me a number of times that she had prayed, asking God to allow her to see her three sons raised into adults. God did grant her that wish as I was 27, my older brother 30, and my younger brother 24 at the time of her crossing.

My mother's last coherent day—before the cancer moved into her brain—I spent a few hours with her at the hospital alone. We talked about life, and the challenges of my youth. She shared with me some secrets from her childhood and early marriage, and we laughed and cried together. Then she told me she was ready to cross over to the other side. She was ready for the mansion God had prepared for her. One of her favorite scriptures was John 14:2: "In my Father's house are many mansions: if it were not so, I would have told you. I go to prepare a place for you." She hung on to this verse through the years of ravaging cancer and the challenges that she faced.

Even though I had her for 17 additional years from what I was told as a child, I was still devastated and angry at God for taking her when he did. My mother, who had never said a bad word about anyone, who served the less fortunate despite her own sickness, who even took in a woman who had been arrested for prostitution while on drugs and subsequently lost her child to the courts. My parents took her in and helped her get her life back by finding housing and even furnishing the apartment so that she could petition the court for her daughter to be returned. She had endured so much—so, so much. And my thoughts were *why or how could a loving God take my wonderful mother, who loved so many people and so many people loved her?* I couldn't understand why.

My mother was a dear soul who had struggled for many years; this was the final straw, the nail in the coffin of my belief or attempt to believe in a loving God. I remember thinking that if there is a

God, he is angry and mean spirited and I would have nothing to do with him. How could he force someone to live their life as if each day might be the last?

The strange thing is how I ended up years later in a similar predicament as my mother. I was living with a time bomb in my chest, and each new day could be my last. I just didn't know the severity of it at the time. If I had, maybe I would not have checked myself out of the hospital in Holland.

— 4 —

"Your Aorta is Torn"

Despite cautions and protests by the hospital personnel, my friend came for me at the hospital in Holland. I was glad to be out. The next couple of days I spent in Holland resting, but also going for long walks to build up my heart muscle, because the diagnosis from the hospital was some type of muscle fatigue while swimming. They felt prescription blood thinners and exercise should do the trick. Yes, prescription blood thinners and exercise. And I was good with that diagnosis. It sounded a heck of a lot better than what I was thinking—heart attack. Little did I know what lurked inside me.

After a few days of rest with my friends in Delft, I decided it was time to go home to Budapest. Still being in some degree of a weakened state, there was concern about me driving across Europe alone in my car. It was really more than a day's drive, but not quite two days. So I decided I would just sleep in my car at the Austrian border that night, and then continue on the next day into Budapest. Ev made a *HELP* sign out of cardboard, so I could put it in the window if I should need help along the way. And I did sleep at the border in my Mazda 323 by lowering the seat back and reclining. Then I set out again early the next morning. I was so happy and so thankful when I arrived at my Budapest flat. It's amazing how our minds will take refuge from fear with the smallest of comforts. I was home, so I must be fine . However, in the back of my mind, I knew I was kidding myself. I wasn't fine.

The weeks that followed were a bit crazy, as I worked to convince myself and others that the Dutch diagnosis was accurate. I believed I was getting stronger. The reality was much different, though. I was gaining weight. Not muscle mass, but flabby fluid weight and looking mighty pale.

A few weeks after the lake incident, my brother, Ken called from Nashville and said he was going to be in London for business. He wanted our other brother, Allen, and me to join him and spend a few days touring around England, London and Oxford areas, climbing towers and hiking the hills. I said, "Yes, of course!" So I flew to London, where we spent a long weekend touring and climbing. We ate meat pies, deliciously fried fish and chips, famed bangers and mash, topped off with luscious helpings of sticky toffee pudding for dessert. I am not a beer drinker, so I did avoid a bit of dead calories and fat, but I struggled often on the climb up those wonderful old church spiral steps. Often too winded to continue and having to take little breaks concerned me. Ken made me promise to see another doctor once I returned to Budapest. I agreed, of course, but with no real plans of following through.

When I left my brothers in England, I flew back across the Channel to Amsterdam. I trained to Delft for a concert with Dave and Ev and a *Tramps* band of Dutch friends that Dave had put together. Dave and Ev were moving back to his home state of Florida, and this would likely be *Morgan & The Tramps* farewell to Europe concert.

We performed on the famed Town Square in front of City Hall, one of the most photographed buildings in Holland. On Saturday evening, we did a full concert of our street music ranging from "California Dreamin'," to "Takin It to The Streets," "Long Train Runnin," "Mrs. Robinson"… lots of great old vocal songs. We had a nice crowd of friends and passersby attendance as it had been advertised in the *Delftse Post* newspaper that week. The following day, after the concert I trained to Amsterdam and flew back to Budapest.

Back in Budapest, I was growing more concerned about my health. I was experiencing weight gain and fatigue. I had a gnawing feeling of fear while on bike rides to and from the office which had a few hills to climb. Sometimes while riding, I would feel the same burning sensation in the middle of my back, which alarmed me. I knew something wasn't right.

Hal Young cornered me after church on Sunday and politely informed me that I was going to see a doctor the next day. Hal and I had been good friends for years by that time, and I was a groomsman and sang in his and Brenda's wedding just a couple of years prior in Atlanta. He was a football coach by training and though mild mannered generally, he told me that I could either go see a doctor on my own, or he would pick me up and carry me. I knew that he meant that literally. Since Hal and I had a Hungarian pastor friend, Mézes Llazlo, who was married to a cardiologist, it was decided that I should go see his wife.

The next day I went to see Dr. Marozsán Ibolya at the Cardiology Hospital. With more than a little hesitation that morning, I dressed and headed out on my trek to the clinic on the Buda side in downtown Budapest. I took the metro under the city arriving at the at Déli Pályaudvar (South Station). I then walked the last few blocks to the beautiful old Austrian-Hungarian stone facade Semmelweis University Heart and Vascular Centre. After informing them that I was there to see Dr. Marozsán, I was directed to sit in the waiting area. On a normal day, sitting in a reception area—whether waiting at the bank or for a ticket to be issued for the train—there was not much apprehension. Thankfully, I did not have to wait long before Dr. Marozsán came for me herself, ushering me back to an examination room. She listened with her stethoscope, and then told me to remove my shirt and lie on my side on the examination table. In front of me was an ultrasound machine. She greased up the wand and began moving it around the center of my chest, pushing and probing as far under my ribcage as was possible. Nothing hurt, and she was smiling, so I began to relax. All of a sudden, she inhaled a sharp breath and said something in Hungarian to a technician close by. She kept the wand in the same place. Moving it ever so slightly, a bit at a time, while my fear escalated. What had she seen? What had she said? She then made another slight gasp, but this time with exclamation in her voice. A few moments later, the door opened, and another doctor appeared. She talked with the doctor and the technicians in somewhat hushed tones in rapid fire Hungarian, and then handed the wand to the visiting doctor who sat and began probing as well. With his face within 24 inches of my face I locked my eyes on his. Then his expression changed as well, and he glanced into my eyes ever so briefly, and then looked back at the screen again, changing his expression to a slight smile, as if to reassure me.

I had been quiet until that moment, allowing them to converse in their intense-sounding Hungarian dialogue. I summoned the courage to ask, "What's going on?"

Ibolya sat back down on the stool and her demeanor changed to that of a mother, a friend, a messenger sent to deliver bad news with warmth and care. She said to me in her English, "Rendi, this is very bad." She paused. "You have a tear in your aorta that must be repaired immediately." She went on to explain the procedure as best she could in her second or third language, English, and I understood all I needed to. I thought, *Am I am going to die?*

She told me to get my shirt on, and then she walked me out into a long sterile cool hallway with white walls, high ceilings, and tiled flooring. She motioned for me to sit on a straight back bench in that hallway. She once again took on the motherly sound of comfort and concern. She told me that she must go now and prepare for the surgery. It would take a bit of time to get everything together, including calling in surgeons and other personnel. She calmly instructed me to sit there and wait. I nodded. I couldn't even muster a question. I watched her walk away.

I remember saying to God, "How can this be true? Have I not served you? Did I not leave home and follow a calling to work for you in the world? Isn't this worth something to you? Is this the best we can do?" I was hurt and somewhat angry about finding myself in this scary place, far from home, so far, so, so far, and even farther from any peace.

I sat watching people walking past me. My mind began to play a video of the faces of my friends and family back home in Nashville. My entire life began to flash or play in my mind. I remember two nurses walking by me in their white lab coats and white clogs and the smell of nicotine and smoke hit me like a brick. Then panic set in. I stood almost instinctively and began to walk. I walked down the hallway towards the entrance and quickly exited the building at a fast pace. Városmajor Park was just a block away from the hospital and I entered that park seeking refuge from the reality that I had just experienced. The large old trees created a canopy of foliage above my head and that seemed to bring me comfort. I tried to sit down on a park bench, but soon realized that I was too panicked to sit. Almost as if I was being hunted. I quickly walked through the park, heading toward the entrance that led back to the metro station in which I had arrived earlier that morning. Once I entered the busy South Station, I started to navigate the steps, sidestepping my way around the hordes of people down below the city where the train cars speed in and out. Then I stopped. Going beneath the city was like entering a tomb. The metros of Budapest were super-efficient, and I used them every day for years, but not that day. I decided I must stay above ground, because as long as I stayed above ground, I was alive.

I crossed the street to the tram stop and soon saw a trolley coming to collect me and the others waiting. As the doors opened, I saw the packed tram cars. Normally I would just push and force my way in like everyone else, but, again, not this day. The thought of collapsing on the streetcar—crammed in with all of those people—made me rethink taking the trolley. So I began a long walk across the city of Budapest.

A few hours later, I was somewhere in the center—most of that walk and the routing of that walk remain unclear to this day. I was in shock. Propelled by fear. I thought of my mother and those nightmares where I couldn't help her. I felt that helpless, but this time I was the center of the nightmare. And I just wanted to live longer, live healthier, be more alive. My life couldn't end like this, so far from home. My walking felt like control. I had to keep moving.

Sometime early to mid-afternoon, I was walking down Ándrassy út, a prominent boulevard on the Pest side of the city. The Buda side has all the hills, and the Pest side is the flatland, and historically the farmlands, the gates to the plains, the breadbasket of Europe.

I had been walking for hours by this time and just decided to stop and see my young friend Fabian Zsolt. I had known Zsolt since the winter of '94 when I had lost my wallet on the street in front of my apartment house. I had been out early that morning and did not even realize that I had lost my wallet until I heard my doorbell ring. I opened the door to find this young man, with his bright smile asking if I had lost the wallet that he was holding. He had found my ID inside and just started asking people on the street if they knew an American man who lived in the area. Expats, *expatriate* as we are called, which I have always thought sounds negative. That is what they call you when you leave your homeland to live in another country. So expats were pretty rare in the early 1990s in Hungary so it didn't take Zsolt long to locate the American man living on Keleti Károly utca, the street where he worked. Zsolti and I became good friends, and I have enjoyed the hospitality of his parents' and grandparents' homes a number of times through the years. Zsolti was the first person I had told of my diagnosis that day roaming through Budapest, but not long after leaving his office I ran into longtime friends Ron and Bonny (Kingsbury) Thiesen at Kodály Körönd Square. We had been working together in ministry since the summer of 1990 in Amsterdam and were close, and remain close friends to this day. They were immediately concerned and supportive as they prayed for me there on the street.

After seeing them I continued my walk down the boulevard, through Városliget (City Park), and szécheny Fürdö (thermal baths) by Mexikói út Metro station, and eventually on to Zugló, to my flat which overlooked Újvidék tér (park) on Szugló utca. Upon entering my flat, later afternoon by this time, I noticed my answering machine, (remember those?) was blinking. The first message was Dr. Marozsán at the hospital in a panic tone asking where I was and if I was okay . Then there was a message from my YWAM friends and colleagues, Hal Young and Steve Johnson. Then, much to my surprise, a couple of calls from the States looking for me as well. It seems that when I disappeared hours before, Dr. Marozsán had called Hal Young, and they began searching for me. Though I do not remember when or where, at some point, after fleeing the hospital, I called my insurance agent friend in Nashville and left a message asking his opinion whether my health insurance would cover surgery in Hungary. This part is a blur, but I do know that my friend Kirk had heard the message when he awoke that morning, as Nashville is seven hours behind Hungary. He tried to call me back to no avail, so he called my brothers and some friends asking if they had heard from me. There was enough concern going around that day on both continents. Eventually, I began returning calls and assuring everyone that I was alive. I called Dr. Marozsán, and explained to her that I had panicked. She said she understood but then told me that I needed to get back to the hospital, immediately. I told her that I wanted to go home to America. Home to Nashville. She said there was no way that she could allow me to fly in my present condition. She said I needed open-heart surgery immediately to repair the tear in my aorta. Flying back to Nashville seemed impossible to her and to me, and yet, for me having surgery there did not seem possible either. She said it was too dangerous, and that I might not survive the flights. I wasn't sure what to do. I am sure that I must have apologized to her for disappearing, but I honestly do not remember. I do remember telling her that I needed some time to think and to pray.

That evening our team met for our usual Monday evening prayer time at the home of Steve and Barbara Johnson, a few blocks away from my apartment. I was the center of the prayers that evening, with lots of love and care as we prayed for healing and for wisdom regarding the next step. After the prayer time ended, Steve offered to take me home and stay with me that night at my flat; he did not want me to be alone. I thanked him but he had a family and I was sure I would be fine through the night. I had to keep reminding myself, and others, that even though I had just heard this diagnosis, I had had this tear for over 8 weeks. I did, however, stop taking the prescription blood thinners immediately, as per Ibolya's instructions!

The following day was Tuesday. I spent the morning trying to gather information about surgery and my chances in order to make a decision to have the operation there or try to get home. I met with an American doctor who was in Budapest for meetings about opening an American Clinic there, and he agreed to meet with me.

After he heard that I had already survived over eight weeks since the original dissection, he agreed that my best outcome would be to get home and have the surgery in my own city and country.

After that conversation I called Ibolya and she was adamant that I would not survive the trip. "You must have surgery here," she said. She could not let me get on a plane.

At that point I changed my approach and I appealed to her as to a mother. I knew her son Áron from times at their church, so I said, "Ibolya, if Áron was in another country and he had a life-threatening issue, but had already survived eight weeks, what would you tell him?"

Silence. Then she said, "I would tell him to come home."

With a shaky voice and through tears, I said, "I must go home."

She then stopped telling me that I *could not* and started telling me what I must do to survive the flights. "You must rest all you can on the plane," then she wrote me a prescription for Valium.

— 5 —

"You Will Never Amount to Anything"

From my earliest memory, I wanted to learn to play the piano. I was fascinated by my neighbor's piano. I loved seeing her fingers gliding across the ivory keys and the beautiful music it created. Sometime during my early elementary school years, I talked my mother into letting me take piano lessons. Someone told my mother about a piano teacher a few streets over from us who was on my walking route home from school. Her huge black grand piano sat in the front room. She was kind but all business. After a few weeks, she told my mother that I needed a piano if I wanted to continue, because I was learning quickly and needed to practice regularly. She thought I had natural ability, which excited me. But it did not translate into excitement for my father. He said we simply could not afford a piano. Then he said, "Pianos are for girls; sports and working on cars are for boys." I am sure money was tight for us, but I believe the real reason was the former. Girls played the piano. And that was that. No one crossed my father, and his decisions were usually final. But my inability to fix things, my lack of confidence to play any sports outside of our backyard basketball goal, and my open desire to play the piano and sing, yes, perform, horrified my father. Maybe it had something to do with surviving the Great Depression in America, seeing poverty firsthand. Men needed jobs to provide for their families. I think he feared that I might follow my heart and my crazy artistic dreams and starve in the process. Feeding the family was the high priority, and he felt you couldn't do it in the music business or having an acting career. All of this may have played a part, but I think he was ashamed of my artistic nature. He viewed me as a *sissy kid* and often said so. We were in church every time the doors were opened, and I heard all about God creating us, the Parable of the Talents, and yet everything that I had natural aptitude, and wanted to do, was wrong. I wondered why this God, who had created a beautiful world with talented people, could have made such a mistake with me. Why was the piano so bad for a boy? I saw male piano players on the television like the *Ed Sullivan Show*. They seemed to enjoy their talents. These feelings of being 'wrong', feeling 'less' or worse, being a '*sissy*' created shame in me and that is possibly when I began building my *wall of humor*.

That wall became a fortress around my heart that served as an impenetrable shield to hide my shame. If I could laugh at myself or make fun of myself before someone else did, it lessened the sting of their remarks, whether jokingly or with malice. I tried hard to never allow myself to show embarrassment, fear, self-doubt or pain. Sadly, I also became skilled at making fun of others to make myself feel better about me, something that I regret to this day. I wish I could go back and apologize to everyone who was hurt or embarrassed by my comments. In the Bible, James 3:6 cautions us, "The tongue also is a fire, a world of evil among the parts of the body." Though my humor has opened doors for me, especially living in a number of foreign countries and communicating without a common language, many times, many places, I have used my humor to connect with people. My quick wit and sense of humor have definitely been two of my greatest assets and yet I, have used these as a wall to keep people out. I regret that.

Looking back, I think my father also had a wall of humor. He used humor at church and with extended family, and he could be fun with us at home as well. Once I was away from home and began to mature and understand myself better, I was also able to understand my father better. As an adult, I learned more about my father's challenging upbringing, which helped me understand his negative behavior and control issues. He was often a hard man to please. But he had a soft side that he often kept hidden. I think his need to hide came from fear of being out of control, like a good portion of his early years. He was born into a family of four—his parents and two older sisters in 1916 during World War I. Within the next four years his mother, Callie Allen-Morgan had another son and a daughter before passing away with my father by her bedside. He was five years old. How devastating and sad this must have been for him. During that era, being the eldest boy came with responsibility to *man-up* and help the family. I'm sure it weighed on my father, as he did his best to help his father and two older sisters work to feed and provide for the two younger ones in those years before the Great American Depression. With five children and with no wife, my grandfather had to place my father and his siblings into an orphanage for a few years. I am unsure which siblings were eventually taken by relatives as babies or by the older girls to serve in relatives' households cooking and cleaning to pay their board. I do know that my father's early life was not easy. Though he did not talk about those years and I cannot prove it or to what level, but I believe he was abused in the orphanage.

Growing up under the *discouragement* of my father, he often told me that I would "never amount to anything." Looking back, I think someone had told him this when he was a boy, and he lived under that lie during his teen years and through his 20s. His behavior changed when he met my mother in his early 30s and married at 32. Sadly, my father was full of shame and carried that shame throughout his life. He wanted his three boys to survive and thrive, but he did not know how to encourage us. Maybe he thought reverse psychology was motivational, but it was not. When you are told you will never amount to anything long enough, you struggle to amount to anything.

A few years after my grandmother Callie Allen died, my grandfather remarried. Papa was able to get all five of his children back under one roof. I can only imagine how my father felt that day returning home after his nightmare. I wonder if he felt bitter toward his father or blamed himself for having to live away from his family. I'm sure the death of his mother and having to live in an orphanage scarred him to some degree. Later Papa's second wife, the only grandmother I knew on the Morgan side, (whom we called Mama Morgan) would have four children of her own, creating a blended home of nine children in all. I know from family stories that was not without its challenges.

My father was thirteen years old when America entered the Great Depression in 1929. The economy started to rebound a bit by 1933 but the Depression continued until America entered World War II in 1941. To add to my father's negative self-image, when called up for military service he was declined after his medical physical due to weakened lungs that he had suffered since birth. His parents were told in his early years that they should not expect him to live through his teens. After my father's death in 1992 my older brother found an old document showing my grandparents had purchased a life insurance policy on him at an early age for a small amount. Probably enough to cover burial costs at that time.

His being denied military service, I think was devastating to my father and thus his already damaged self-image. His younger brother and two half-brothers went off to war without him. He remained at home with another half-brother who couldn't serve due to polio and was dependent upon leg braces for his entire life. I believe the embarrassment of not being able to serve his country caused him to sink further into self-doubt, self-hatred and anger. This may have started or fortified his own wall of humor.

As a teenager, I believed my father hated me, and I tried to hate him. At times I even told myself that I hated him. But, with most children, our nature is to love our parents, despite the pain and disappointments. Still, I could never do right in his eyes. I remember one evening, as an adult, after my mother had passed, I went over to be with my father for a while and he started into one of his horrible tirades of what a disappointment I was and had been, and I knew it would end badly. So I countered the best I could. I gave him some of my thoughts based on courses from college, but he would not be pacified. His anger grew and he finally said to me, "You have always thought you were smarter than me." That was a light bulb moment. That seemed to be one of his greatest fears, that his sons would be smarter or more successful than he was. Shouldn't a father want their kids to surpass him in everything, including intelligence, career, even parenthood?

In the years since his passing I have come to the belief that his self-image was so bad that maybe he believed in the quiet of his heart that nothing *good* could come from him. My father was a very smart man, but I believe his early life *messages* were so strong and damaging that he was never able to believe in himself. Being completely honest, I am not so sure that I would have done any better had I been in his shoes. My childhood was easy in comparison to his childhood. I do not want anyone reading this to think I am being terribly unfair to my father. This is not my goal. My goal is to help people find hope despite those early messages of life. I know that I am not the only person who had an overbearing negative parent. Sometimes we just have to take a step back and examine their lives, their life messages when they were young. Their circumstances shaped them as ours did us. Sadly, those messages often get passed down through the generations.

I believe with all of my heart that both of my parents crossed over from this life into the arms of Jesus, their Savior. They were both strong believers and though we had more than our share of problems, they did model Christ to me, and I believe if they could come back from across the Great Divide, they would be proud of my wanting to help others by using the positives and negatives of my life. And my parents' investment, both the good and the bad, has resulted in my being able to help others. My parents had a lot to do with my desire and passion to bring hope to the hurting.

One of the most difficult aspects of growing up in a religious home was hearing about how God created us and the mixed message that was for me. I heard that He created us with talents and abilities to be used for His glory. But it seemed to me that everything I wanted to do was *wrong*. I wanted to play music and perform, but being members of the Church of Christ, there were no musical instruments. In the Church of Christ, at that time most, if not all, of the congregations in our area did not believe in using musical instruments because there is no biblical reference of them being used in the first century church. So we should not play them either. I wondered often about other traditions we enjoyed at church that also were not mentioned in the New Testament of the Bible.

I loved and still love a cappella congregational singing. I enjoy hearing the four-part harmonies ringing out, so I didn't grow up thinking we needed an instrument in the service. In our church services, we had a song leader who would be the only mic'd vocal, and he would direct with his hand the meter of the song. I really can't remember ever watching the song leader much. I was too focused on singing the correct notes, whether I was singing the tenor or the alto.

At church camp my friend Joel could play his guitar and we could sing all sorts of popular secular songs and that was fine . It was just confusing for me even as a teenager. That confusion would grow in the years that followed.

If we had a wedding, there had to be special permission to even have a rented piano or organ brought into the church, and often it had to be out of the church before the Sunday service. At my wedding in 1975 at Hillsboro Church of Christ on Hillsboro Road in Nashville, we brought in an organ and a piano and somehow got them to the balcony, but they had to be taken out that night. They were not allowed to even be in the building for the next morning's Sunday service. Why, someone might have passed out or had a heart attack had they seen a piano in the building during a Sunday morning service.

Thinking of heart attacks brought me back to reality very quickly as I continued to roam through Budapest with the weight of my diagnosis on my back.

— 6 —

Angels From Heaven

With my prescription of Valium in hand, I was going to the airport and would do whatever it took to get on that plane that would take me home to Nashville. Ferenc Liszt International Airport, formerly known as Budapest Ferihegy was 10 miles south of downtown Budapest. Steve came for me early that morning and as I turned off the lights and locked the door, I wondered if I would ever return to my flat, my home. After a day and a half of weighing out the odds and tons of prayers from both sides of the ocean, Steve and I went to the airport with determination, even if it meant having to buy a first class ticket. Living on a missionary budget, to buy a first class ticket would be well beyond my funding but I told myself if that was the only seat on the plane, I would purchase that ticket on my credit card and worry about that bill later.

Thankfully a friend who worked at Delta in Atlanta had given me a Buddy Pass a few months earlier which resulted in securing a Business Class seat. Once in the air, the flight attendant came to me and asked the nature of my medical emergency that Steve and I had told the ticket agent. We had *pulled out all the stops* to ensure a seat on the plane. It may have been advantageous at that moment to have lied or at least hedged around the truth, but I decided to tell her the hard reality of my medical situation. I started regretting that decision as soon as it came out of my mouth as her face registered surprise then maybe even shock! She then kindly asked if I had written permission to fly. Written permission? From whom? She said from a doctor. I had not even thought of such a thing, so while praying silently in my mind, I dug out my three Valium tablets in the little plastic bottle with my name, yesterday's date and the name of Dr. Mározsán on the label, hoping that would show approval from my doctor; then the adrenaline rush of the past 40 hours came crashing down, and my eyes filled with tears as I said, "Please, you have to get me home."

She looked deeply into my eyes and eventually replied, "We will get you home."

At that moment, our relationship was sealed. She was an angel sent from heaven and would prove it a few more times before we landed in Atlanta some ten hours later.

In 1997, Delta routed through Frankfurt, Germany for additional passenger pickups, and those on the plane from Budapest did not exit but just stayed on as the new passengers were added. My concern was being put off the plane in Frankfurt now that the airline crew knew the severity of my medical condition. But this flight attendant (the purser on this flight, from what I heard from other attendants) had really gone to bat for me using her knowledge as a nurse to convince the crew that I should stay onboard, and she would keep an eye on me. I learned later that not only was she a trained nurse, but also a committed Christ Follower! Another God-appointed detail.

Once back in the air after our brief stopover in Germany, the purser told me that she had learned there was a team of doctors and nurses on the plane who had been on a mission trip in Romania. She had talked with a couple of those doctors, and soon they began visiting me on a regular rotation through out the long overseas flight, checking my blood pressure, heart rate, and discussing my vitals as I if I were in a room in a hospital. ICU in Business Class… another God-appointed detail.

My only regret is not knowing the names of the Delta purser and the medical staff who attended me on that flight. Once we landed in Atlanta, it was a whirlwind as a Delta representative met me with a wheelchair and fast-tracked me through passport control, and customs. Once I was in the domestic area in Atlanta's airport my very efficient attendant and chair driver explained the next steps in getting me to an ambulance and on to an Atlanta hospital. Wait! I want to go home, home to Nashville!

I started praying silently, and quickly did yet another *song and dance* about getting home to Nashville. In a pleading voice I said I had come so far that *surely* I could make one more short flight to Nashville. A 45-minute flight and I would be home. I had family and friends already waiting at the Nashville airport and medical appointments booked, just a short flight away. To my amazement, it worked! She wheeled me to the gate to board me on to Nashville. Another God-appointed detail.

Oh what joy I felt when those jet wheels hit the tarmac at Nashville International Airport! I was home! Home! Thankful does not adequately explain my feelings. I had friends waiting who scooped me up and took me to their house for a long, Valium-laced sleep. There might be challenges to face ahead, but I was home, I was at peace that The Lord had brought me home.

The next afternoon would be my first cardiology appointment in Nashville. I felt we would get the full story, the correct story. I was feeling confident now. I had survived. God was still faithful.

On Thursday, after a bit of a lie-in, as my British friends say, a couple of friends drove me to a cardiology office located at Saint Thomas Medical Center in Nashville. Upon arrival I was sent directly to a technician who would perform yet another echocardiogram before I would meet the doctor. It was late in the day so it was determined that I should return the following day to meet the cardiologist and learn the results of the test. On Friday morning we returned for me to meet and discuss the test findings with Dr. Glazer. I immediately liked Mark Glazer. He was personable and funny which put me at ease. The best was, he was happy to inform me that his technician had not found any sign of a dissection. Really? The Hungarian doctors were wrong? Ibolya had not seen what she and her colleagues thought they had seen? Dr. Glazer then said it did appear that my aortic valve was not operating correctly; therefore, he wanted to see me back on Tuesday morning for an arteriogram to determine the severity of the situation. I thought, "There you have it. Those Hungarian doctors—bless their hearts. That's what you get with a post-communist country. I am sure that they did their best." I thought all of those things, or was I just telling myself those things because I wanted to believe this latest diagnosis? I honestly was not sure what to believe. I was happy for this latest news even though I was not convinced that Dr. Mározsán and her colleagues could have all been wrong. But hey, I am not a doctor, and so I am going to believe the latest, I am thrilled with the news, let's go with it!

I called my friend Steve that afternoon and informed him of the Nashville doctor's assessment. We rejoiced together on the phone. After our conversation, he phoned Dr. Mározsán, as promised, to tell her the news. But she would not be convinced. She was adamant. She told Steve, "No Steve, I saw it. You tell him to tell those doctors that he has a dissection of the aorta."

Steve called me back to tell me what she had said. *Hmm … who to believe?* I wanted to believe the American and patronize the Hungarian, but… well, anyway the day was over and the weekend upon me. I will just stick my head back in the sand for now. After all, it had been in the sand for a good portion of the last eight weeks. Actually, in some ways, in the sand for most of my childhood and young adult life. I guess my head felt comfortable there.

— 7 —

The Little Suitcase Piano

Sometime prior to my teen years, my mother told me that one of her sisters, Mildred, had called and wanted to give me my cousin Jan's little suitcase piano. I have no memory of her playing the piano, but I have great memories of her father playing. I enjoyed watching him and listening when we would visit their home. I was fascinated by his ability to play, largely by ear. Uncle Robert was a kind, fun uncle, a man, and a member of the Church of Christ and yet, he played the piano and no one appeared upset by that. I wondered why was it so wrong for me?

That electric piano was made into a hard case with a lid that opened on hinges and an electric cord for the wall. It looked like a suitcase. In my memory, it had a three to four-octave keyboard which was less than half the size of a real piano, but it was enough to satisfy my desire to play. I would sit for hours and teach myself chords. I even figured out a bit of my own number system with one being the root, the four and five chords, and you could play a lot of hymns, and even pop songs on chords one, four and five.

Through my teens I escaped to that piano often where I would sit on the floor and play. Then the summer before my senior year of high school, one of my classmates sold me her old upright grand piano for a couple of hundred dollars, and I moved it into our home. Surprisingly, my father didn't seem to mind, or he was just past caring. Maybe he finally realized I would not be one of the *sons* at *Morgan & Sons Electric Company*.

Immediately after graduation from Isaac Litton High School, I went to work for Nashville's Newspaper Printing Corporation. I started at an entry level position delivering advertising "tear sheets" for the Advertising Department of the NPC. This was long before computers, and the larger department stores had in-house artists who drew pictures of women and men in their dresses and suits. Those ads had to be picked up from their art departments and delivered to the NPC Art Department, which also had a large Art Department for all of those advertisers who did not have in-house artists. These drawings and advertising proofs had to be driven over and approved, then returned for another approval once a preliminary drawing had been printed. Driving back and forth on my downtown or Green Hills route, I would have my 8-track portable player on the back seat of my navy blue 1965 Mustang convertible, and would sing along with the Mamas and the Papas, The Eagles, and other vocal band type groups.

After a few months I was offered a new position within the NPC in the accounting department. I began working in the cashiers cage, and one of my duties was getting the payroll checks written, balanced and distributed to over one thousand employees. At 18 years of age, that was a lot of responsibility for me, which helped me gain some confidence.

The newspaper printing machines were extremely loud and they employed many deaf people to work in that area. These deaf employees would come to me in the cashier's cage to get information about their insurance or withholding amounts from their paychecks. I had to learn to communicate with them. Obviously we did most of our communication via pencil and paper, and I started to learn some communication skills beyond my comfort level. I began to notice and value people who were not like me. I also learned that my facial expressions were vital in good communication. These were skills that I would later find useful living in countries where I did not speak the language. A smile goes a long way to disarm and create trust.

I stayed at that job until late summer of 1971, when I decided I wanted to enroll in college. Seems I had taken a *Gap Year* between high school and college which I needed to develop and catch up to my peers. Another of my mother's sisters worked in the Registrar's Office at David Lipscomb College so I called my Aunt Edith and she fast-tracked my paperwork in order for me to start to college in September.

David Lipscomb College, now Lipscomb University, a Church of Christ liberal arts college with a cozy campus in the Green Hills neighborhood of Nashville. Sometime in my first quarter I ran into a high school classmate, Terry Owens. Soon I was commuting daily with Terry and two of his friends from church. They were sisters, Debbie and Dusty Logue. We had a great time in our commutes but were often late, it seemed. One morning we were late for our early class and the professor saw us attempt to sneak in on the back row of the lecture hall, and he immediately called us to the front. He asked us if we remembered the children's song "Building Up the Temple." Though I had not grown up in the same congregation as Terry, we had been raised in similar churches and knew the song, which pleased Dean McKelvey. He asked, "Do you know the hand motions that accompany the song?" We did, of course, but realized quickly that we should have said no. So he had us perform the song along with the hand motions which were fist over fist—building up the temple of the Lord. Though embarrassing, it was also funny, and we laughed probably as much as we sang. Since the large percentage of Lipscomb students at that time came out of the Church of Christ, most of the students knew it as well, though I don't remember anyone singing along. We survived our performance, and it did help us to be more punctual in the weeks to come.

I entered college with the plan to major in art. I had taken art every year in high school and had enjoyed it. I made some great friends during my freshman year in the art department and enjoyed the courses. I also started making friends in the music department and soon a friend convinced me to audition for one of Lipscomb's choruses, The Chorale led by Dr. Gerald Moore. I made the audition and for the next few years sang with the Chorale, but also built a relationship with Dr. Moore. He was a kind and patient man and would become more of a father figure in my life. He was an encourager, which I needed. I had the honor of serving as president of the Chorale for a season, which allowed me a lot of time with him. In recent years he told me that I was welcome to call him Gerald. I just could not; he was too high on my list of life influencers. That season of music connected me more with the music department than the art department. Soon I would change my focus and my major to music. I was asked to join Lipscomb's premier A Capella Chorus a couple of times but declined, but I did eventually sing with Chamber Singers, but I just could not leave Dr. Moore and the Chorale family.

I was part of a number of groups and bands at Lipscomb. One traveled in recruitment for the school as well as performing at Junior/Senior Banquets. These banquets were big in the Church of Christ. Because dancing was greatly feared within 'the church' as a slippery slope into all manner of sin, a number of young people in more conservative homes were not allowed to attend their school proms. Dancing, you know! So a group of churches would host a Junior/Senior Banquet where all the young people from the churches in their area would dress in their formal wear, corsages were purchased and pinned, and off they would go for an evening of food and entertainment.

Country music and the Grand Ole Opry were the last things on my mind as a teenager. When I entered college I was more into pop and early lite rock music. I was a big vocal band person, growing up singing alto and tenor. I loved the sound and intricacies of harmonies such as Peter Paul and Mary, the Kingston Trio, the Everly Brothers, then later with the Supreme's and The Temptations. When they did their big special "Taking Care of Business," I was hooked and mesmerized by every aspect of that show. I still have the LP album. The vocals, the dancing, the colorful 60s outfits, they just had it all.

Country music was not cool in my teenage years, despite Barbara Mandrell's hit single, "I Was Country When Country Wasn't Cool." That may have worked well for Barbara, but wasn't cool for me, nor anyone I knew in my Nashville high school.

Music became my focus and I joined up with two friends, Dianne Corbitt and Larry Lockwood to form, wait for it… Corganwood. Yes, CORbitt/MorGAN/LockWOOD. Seriously, I couldn't make that up. Corganwood performed at the college talent show, then at different campus events, local venues, social clubs, and even at the original O'Charley's restaurant.

Larry Lockwood and I were in the same social club, which was Lipscomb's version of fraternities and sororities. Larry was my roommate in the high-rise dorm. Eight floors made it the tallest building in Green Hills at that time, so it was creatively named High Rise. Larry was and is super smart in math and always maintained a high grade point average in all of his studies. Me? Not so much. We were the *Odd Couple,* a 70s sitcom about two men, fussy photographer Felix and sloppy sportswriter Oscar who end up sharing a New York City apartment. I was neat and preferred social life over studies, and Larry was, hmmm, less than neat, and though social, kept his studies as his priority. Larry finished his studies with a PhD in Statistics, while I struggled with Math 150. However, we are still friends today, and I hope that will continue after he reads this.

After Corganwood, I was asked to sing with Lee Milam, Tom Marcrom and Gary Hale in a quartet we named the Saxons. As a quartet we sang for churches and church events mostly, and soon added Dianne Corbitt, to add to our 'secular' show for the Junior/Senior Banquets. As I have written, the banquets were to provide a place for juniors and seniors in high school to go for dinner and music without dance. Although, at Lipscomb we could dance during stage productions like Singarama, but thankfully God created a loophole called choreography. Choreographed movement was not dancing; therefore it would not draw the eye to sin. Full disclosure, I may have sinned a few times anyway.

One Monday morning, after a weekend away singing, we were called to the Dean's Office at Lipscomb. It seemed that we were reported for singing a sacred song with musical instruments. We were surprised that someone would tell the dean this, and we assured the dean we had not. We had a secular show with instruments and a sacred show that was a cappella for church events. Well, the song in question was "Let There Be Peace on Earth," a song written by Jill Jackson-Miller and Sy Miller in 1955, which has been covered by numerous other artists, including Grand Ole Opry star Vince Gill. It seems that the line *With God as our Father, brothers all are we* was the offending lyric. We were told if we were to sing that song again with instruments, we would need to change that lyric to *With he as our father, brothers all are we*. But we were allowed to sing *God as our father*... a cappella? Really? Seriously? I think at that moment I realized my belief in a God who would care about this was just too weird for me. That marked the beginning of my journey away from church, away from God, away from the traditions of my childhood. I was lost. I had basically learned all the motions and jumped through all the hoops of church as I saw it, but I was done.

After singing together in the Lipscomb Chorale, the bands *Corganwood*, and the *Saxons*, in 1975 Dianne and I were married at Hillsboro Church of Christ. We had been traveling and singing together for a few years, were good friends and had deep affection for each other. We were "cute together" according to others, and it was kind of understood in my church group that you went to Lipscomb to find a Church of Christ spouse. So despite concerns and even some counsel, I asked if she would marry me, and she said, "Yes."

Lee Milam was always finding the music and songs that we would sing. We were a full-harmony vocal band that had a secular show and a sacred show for a cappella churches. One of the bands that we covered was country sensation, Dave and Sugar. Dave and Sugar did a lot of love songs and enjoyed peak success in the mid-to-late 1970s.

The Saxon's also covered a few songs from a Grand Ole Opry group, The Four Guys who in the late 60s had toured with country greats like Faron Young, Jimmy Dean and Charlie Pride. This was one of my first introductions to singing country, pop music. Later, the four of them would open a Nashville night club, dinner theatre called The Four Guys' Harmony House. A male quartet singing "Shenandoah" and a number of just good four-part harmony songs. So as we did more country-pop, I began to warm to country music. On a fun side note, sometime around 1980, *The Four Guys* lost their high tenor, and I went to the Harmony House and auditioned with the guys. After singing their music through the 70s while at Lipscomb, it was a fun few hours singing with them in person. I remember their encouragement after the first song when one of them said, "Oh man, a real tenor." I had a great and fun audition but in the end they hired Laddie Cain, who had nightclub experience which I did not. At least that's what Brent Burkett and Sam Wellington said to me afterwards. They were probably correct. I'm not sure I was ready for a nightclub environment, but I had a great time singing with those *four guys* at the audition.

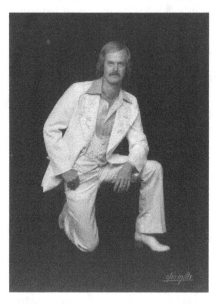

At Lipscomb, I became close friends with Debbie Logue who worked for the Grand Ole Opry after college. She took over the stage managing from Ann Cooper, who was known as Opry Annie. Opry Annie had been raised just one street over from our house, but I did not know her until I started visiting Debbie at the Opry House. Debbie became the secretarial assistant to Hal Durham, who was the manager of the Opry. By the mid to late 70s, I was at the Grand Ole Opry often. Debbie always invited me to hang out with her on her bench on the Friday or Saturday night Grand Ole Opry shows. I spent a lot of weekends hanging out with Debbie and getting to know the Opry family backstage. One of Debbie's responsibilities was being at every Opry performance to keep track of the musicians and artists, so the payroll could be figured and distributed. I spent many Friday and/or Saturday nights on Debbie's two-seater bench. All the artists would enter from backstage just behind that podium curtain and next to Debbie's bench. It was backstage and in the Green Room and the dressing rooms that I got to know many of these true icon Opry Stars. Legends like Bill Monroe, Roy Acuff, Minnie Pearl, Jack Greene, Bill Monroe, Little Jimmy Dickens, and so many more. Every performer and his or her band was assigned to a dressing room. These were large rooms with an additional lounge area that offered coffee and other refreshments backstage. Mr. Acuff's room was always full of people, some friends, some performers, some guests of performers that came to meet the stars. Mr. Acuff was always the perfect host and absolutely loved The Opry and its people.

Often during the evening there would be spontaneous music that would just happen in these dressing rooms. Just a bunch of pickers and singers who would jam together. One of those evenings I remember joining in singing harmony with Billy Walker. One of Billy's hit records was "Cross the Brazos at Waco," a country western ballad. Billy told me that evening about his giving up his seat on the Randy Hughes private plane and returning on a commercial flight due to a family need. That flight would eventually take off with Patsy Cline, Cowboy Copas, Hawkshaw Hawkins, and manager and pilot Randy Hughes. Sadly, the plane crashed about 100 miles outside of Nashville in a forest near Camden, TN. Though country music was not attractive to me, Patsy Cline had crossed over and I had seen her on the *Arthur Godfrey Show*. I still remember being in the car with my mother on the way to school when I heard on the radio that Patsy Cline had been killed in a plane crash.

Mr. Acuff loved my friend Debbie, and when she adopted her first child, Julia, Mr. Acuff passed her car—one afternoon walking back to his house—and thought, *She can't drive her baby around in that car.* So later that afternoon he brought her thousands of dollars in cash and told her to go out and get a new car. Mr. Acuff was a generous man and loved his Opry family.

Every thirty minutes, the curtain came down at the Opry, and the sponsor would change from sponsors like Goo Goo Clusters, Dollar General Stores, to Cracker Barrel, Purina Dog Chow, and many more. There was a sponsor for every thirty-minute segment. One evening the curtain was about to go up on the Purina Dog

Chow Show and the curtain would not budge. The motor was running but the curtain was not moving. The music had begun but the curtain was still down. Now, this was a huge heavy curtain, and the Opry stage is no small stage. But someone had the idea to get a bunch of people out there to pick up the curtain and shoulder it on their shoulders so at least the show *could* and *must* go on. I just remember that the announcer behind Debbie's bench had begun the Purina portion advertisement and one of the guys holding the curtain started to bark. Others immediately joined in, and there was the symphony of barking, which tickled the announcer, and he could hardly get the words out. The audience was laughing, everyone was laughing. That type of family feel was not uncommon backstage at the Opry. A great bunch of down-to-earth people who just loved to *pick and sing* coming together to do the show. A family. The Opry family. And I am proud that I had a small place in that family.

Are You a Patient?

Though I was unsure and unsettled by the conflicting reports on my health, I was still at home in Nashville. I was excited to see friends and family in the days ahead. After all the drama of the past weeks and the emergency flight home, I was just glad to be home and at least hopeful that my diagnosis was not as bad as previously believed. I was just focused on enjoying the weekend. I was staying with friends, Bob and Pat Kernodle in Brentwood, just south of Nashville. On Sunday morning other friends, Brett and Erin Barry came to collect me to take me to their church for prayer. All the prayer and the messages of prayer were so encouraging and appreciated. I was still getting messages of concern and prayer from all over the globe, and this was even before social media came into existence.

Despite jet lag, the weekend was nice, but short. I had to deal with the problem at hand, which hung over my head leading me into Tuesday morning all too quickly. It was an early appointment at Saint Thomas Medical Center so I was up very early. Pat drove us to the hospital a bit before 6:00 am. When we arrived in the Imaging Reception, there was no one behind the desk. It was early and maybe they had just stepped away, so we sat down in the waiting area.

We were the only ones seated in the waiting area, and yet there were lots of medical personnel in scrubs coming in and out, some grabbing coffee, and there were even donuts on a table. After a few minutes a nurse came to us and sat down to explain all the commotion. She was Billy Clark, head nurse and leader of the Saint Thomas Hospital Cath Lab at that time. She presumed that we were waiting there for a friend or family member who had already been called back and prepped for an arteriogram. She explained that Saint Thomas was producing a documentary-style commercial series, and a number of these people in scrubs were part of a film crew. It seems they were interviewing and watching to find just the right case to follow for their project. My friend Pat, said to Billy motioning her head over to me, "Well, this is who you should be filming."

At that moment, Billy said, "Oh, are you a patient?" I had still not been registered as a patient so she had no idea. Billy immediately got me called back and into a room in the pods. Somewhere in that process, probably while I was changing into a hospital gown, Pat told Billy the harrowing story of my diagnosis in Budapest and the journey home. Billy, in turn, went to the director of the team and told her the story. The director, who by the way was the double Academy Award-winning Barbara Kopple. Ms. Kopple had won two Academy Awards; the first in 1976 for *Harlan County, USA*, about a Kentucky miners' strike,and the second in 1991 for *American Dream*, the story of the 1985–86 Hormel strike in Austin, Minnesota.

Once I was tucked in to my little gurney-bed in my not-so-lovely gown, Billy came to tell me that Ms. Kopple was interested in meeting me. Almost immediately Barbara Kopple came into the room and explained to me that she and her team were there to film a patient who was having bypass surgery. From this footage, they hoped to create commercials that would hopefully reduce fear in men, and women, who were notorious avoiders and procrastinators when it came to seeing a heart doctor, even when they might be experiencing symptoms. Yes, I could relate.

According to Barbara, they had been following a number of potential cases with some Saint Thomas heart doctors and had planned over a couple of days to pick one that they could follow and film through their entire procedure. Diagnosis to recovery. They brought their crew in from New York and other places around the States to monitor these cases and these doctors from the first step *'Diagnosis'* in the Cath Lab—to see which one would be best to follow. One of the cases turned out to be going home when the arteriogram revealed nothing in the way of blockage. A second man had declined being filmed when he realized they would follow him every day with cameras on him 24-7. The third potential patient did not seem to talk very much, and they were concerned about getting enough dialogue. Well, those of you who know me know that talking would certainly not be a problem, which was a fact Pat quickly pointed out to Barbara and Billy.

Would I agree to them filming my arteriogram? "Sure, of course, let*'s do it*", but it certainly became something much bigger than just filming that one test.

— 9 —

A Big Grand Ole Opry Welcome...

After college my wife and I, along with another couple, bought an old fixer-upper house built in 1889 by a riverboat captain. It was told to us by some of the older neighbors that he had built the corner house for his wife who was confined to a wheel chair. She could be wheeled out on to the Victorian wrap-around porch and visit with the passersby. Inside the big old house we had separate bedrooms and sitting rooms, but joint kitchen and bathroom. We were young and had just left dorm life at Lipscomb, so living together, sharing space was just more of the same. The first year was great fun despite the extreme cold draft of the uninsulated house. But spring would come quickly, and with spring, came a new season with careers taking off. The house project became more work and effort than fun. So I sold my half to the other couple, and we moved down the street and purchased a 1920s bungalow that required far less work.

There were a number of houses in East Nashville undergoing renovations at that time and we eventually had the area zoned historic and protected under the name "Historic Edgefield". A couple of blocks away from us was one such house on Russell Street. It was being renovated by Bill Wade, originally from the state of Maine. Bill, a converted southerner, was the president of Briggs Paint Manufacturing on Woodland Street just a couple of blocks over. One day, while socializing in the neighborhood, Bill asked me to come to work for him. Though my wife and I were singing and doing gigs as often as we could, I needed a job and readily took him up on his offer. I started at the front counter mixing paint and learning about mixing custom colors. Soon I was promoted to Bill's Administrative Assistant. I was learning more about the business end of paint manufacturing and sales, while helping to develop the Decorating Center.

One afternoon, a gentleman came into the store asking for a decorator to help him with a rather large project in one of Nashville's downtown office buildings. Well, both of our decorators were out of the building on other jobs. Bill quickly came to me and told me to get down there and help this gentleman. I had no decorating experience but had been an art major in high school and in college, for a time, and had always enjoyed colors and creativity. So I went to meet the customer. After my spending some time with him, he liked my ideas. Thus, my decorating career was born. Soon I was bidding other jobs and wore two hats—Administrative Assistant and part-time Designer.

Bill was a motivator and loved to encourage his staff just as he had done with me. One day he scheduled all of the sales staff and upper management to attend a conference in Nashville where I heard motivational speaker Zig Ziglar speak for the first time. I was blown away by his delivery and positive attitude for life. Being raised in somewhat of a negative environment, I was hungry for positivity. I wanted to believe in myself, not just pretend I was positive. Zig was full of stories of success and passion. He sure came off as the real deal. I remember that Zig had said, in one of his talks, that he was just passing on what he had learned in the Bible.

It wasn't long after this conference that I learned that our piano-playing friend, Janet McMahan, was writing some of Zig's favorite stories and characters into songs. Janet was helping to create some music that reflected his messages. She called my wife and me about singing on some demo tracks for Zig's motivational music. We went into the studio and recorded a number of songs like "There's a Giant Living Inside You," "Today Is the First Day of the Rest of Your Life," and Dianne soloed on "See You at The Top", which was the title of one of Zig's most popular books.

Soon after the recording session, my wife flew to Dallas with Janet to sing "See You at The Top" for one of Zig's conferences. I flew out and joined them at some point, and we spent some time with the Ziglar Corporation staff, and I was hooked. I wanted to be part of this organization. While I was in Texas I had spoken with Zig about my desire to organize the Zig Ziglar Singers who could perform with him at Ziglar events, Amway and Mary Kay conventions as well. He was very receptive to the idea so almost immediately I returned to Nashville, to my job at Briggs. After sharing this with my friend and boss, Bill, I resigned my position and closed up our house in Edgefield and moved us to Dallas, Texas.

Janet introduced us to her friends, the Peavys. In addition to Wayne's dental practice and Linda's design projects, the couple owned an upscale Mexican restaurant in North Dallas, located in Carillon Towers next to the Valley View Mall. Alaman's had delicious food, recipes mostly created by Linda. Since the owners lived in Arlington, which was more than an hour journey through the Dallas traffic, they needed a general manager who could meet people well, remember names, basically *work the room*. After a few visits, they decided I could be that person. When Wayne called to ask me if I would take the job, I said I had only worked at Mc-Donald's when I was *16*—for one week. He assured me I would not be waiting tables but overseeing the staff and managing. But, mainly, maintaining the clientele. There were a number of well-known patrons of Alaman's including the Ziglar family, a number from the Dallas Cowboy football team, including, Roger and Marianne Staubach.

I immediately loved Alaman's and the vibe of the restaurant business. I also loved being around the Ziglar Corp people and making plans for a full time singing group. My wife was doing weekend gigs with Zig and I was able to attend and enjoy a few of those conferences.

A few months into our move to Dallas, I flew home to Nashville to see my parents and found my mother was not doing well. She wasn't healing from the breast cancer surgery and getting weaker. On the flight back to Texas I knew that I needed to move us back to Nashville. Within the next few days I told the Peavys that I would be leaving the restaurant and then met with Zig to tell him that we would be moving home to be with my mother, for whatever time she had left. They were all gracious and in agreement with my decision. My wife and I returned to Nashville in spring of 1980. We had only been gone less than half a year and we still had our Boscobel Street home in Historic Edgefield.

My wife auditioned and was hired by Grand Ole Opry legend Jim Ed Brown. Jim Ed had an industry breakup with vocal duet partner, Helen Cornelius. Jim Ed's manager, Tandy Rice, and successful management company, Top Billing, came up with the plan to partner Jim Ed with two younger women—my wife, Dianne and Christy Russell. This would make Jim Ed's engagements more like the original Browns. Jim Ed had started his career with his sisters, Maxine and Bonnie, as The Browns. As time passed Maxine and Bonnie either lost interest in the music business, or they had families to raise so they left the stage life. Jim Ed went out on his own and sometime in the late 1970s his label matched him up with female singer Helen Cornelius. Jim Ed and Helen started turning out hits and won the CMA Vocal Duet of The Year Award for their 1976 hit, "I Don't Want to Have to Marry You." Unfortunately, Jim Ed and Helen made some bad decisions with their personal relationship, which brought an end to their professional duet arrangement and left Jim Ed back in a solo career. Teaming him up with two young ladies was the perfect solution and he continued to tour and work the Grand Ole Opry regularly.

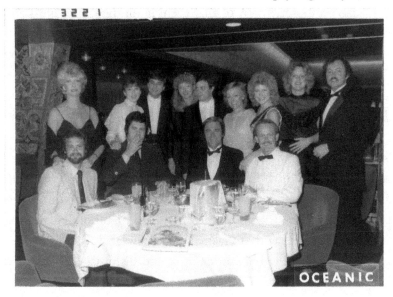

Jim Ed Brown, band and spouses, SS Oceanic

Backstage at the Opry there was often singing and jamming that would break out in one dressing room or another. Jim Ed and I had sung together backstage at the Opry a number of times, so one weekend when his singer Christy had to go home to Oklahoma for a family issue, he asked if I wanted to fill in the third harmony on that Opry weekend. I was definitely happy to do so. I knew all their music and as a first tenor, my range was high enough to cover the lower female part. It is one of the highlights of my music career the evening Jim Ed Brown introduced me, "First time on the Grand Ole Opry, please give a big Opry welcome to Randy Morgan." (I went by Randy at that time.) Jim Ed, Dianne, and I sang a number of his hits that evening but the most famous was "The Three Bells," also known as "Little Jimmy Brown," a song made popular by The Browns in 1959. It was originally a Swiss song *"Les trois cloches,"* written in French by Jean Villard Gilles. The lyrics were adapted to English by Dutch artist, Bert Reisfeld.

I have a cassette copy of that evening on the Opry, and I still enjoy an occasional listen to our trio version of "The Three Bells".

A lot of weekends were spent backstage at The Opry. There were shows on Friday and two shows on Saturday evening. Between shows we would drive over to The Nashville Palace on Music City Drive. It was a dinner club and bar that would have live music and often had a house band. Jim Ed's band would go over and often share a song or two. The Nashville Palace was managed by Lib Hatcher from North Carolina. Lib had moved to Nashville with fellow Carolinian, Randy Traywick, who would sing under the name Randy Ray. Lib and Randy both had high hopes of getting him a record deal with a Nashville country label. Randy worked in the kitchen as a short order cook and dishwasher. He would often come out and sing a solo or two and we became friends. Eventually, Randy got a recording deal with Warner Brothers, they changed his name to Randy Travis, and the rest is history. Our paths continued to cross over the next few years.

— 10 —

Do You Want to Star in a Television Docu-Drama?

While in my hospital room, despite these being potentially my darkest hours, I enjoyed the banter with the film crew. They were with me during the arteriogram and filmed the cardiologist delivering his assessment that there could actually be a tear in my aorta. So there you have it!

It seemed that for Barbara Kopple, it was decided. I was the one she would film, but she ended up having to fight hard. I heard a good portion of a heated discussion between her, the surgeon, Dr. Petracek, Kevin Endres of Endres Wilson Advertising Agency, and the hospital CEO.

The pods were very close together with paper-thin walls separating them. Evidently when the surgeon was called in and learned that Barbara Kopple and her team would be filming this surgery, he was not happy. Only feet away from me—out of sight, but not out of earshot—an argument ensued. I was listening to the doctor explain in full volume, that my case was too risky. He listed a number of things that would make this a bad idea, including my death, being permanently paralyzed, unable to speak or see.

This was not very comforting. The picture was bleak at best. He was simply not comfortable filming my case. The CEO—knowing the risks they would be taking: the costs involved and with an Academy Award winning director and film crew—understood the liabilities if I was unable to film the smiling conclusion. All of the film and days of labor would be lost, and they would be back to square one without a commercial series, not to mention all the money lost.

I learned much later that an emergency meeting was called of the Saint Thomas Hospital Board of Directors to discuss the pending filming, possibly 'pulling the plug' on the commercials. I do not know who presented the case to the Board, but in the end, Ms. Kopple was quite persuasive and won the support of the hospital's CEO, convincing the Board that this was the right case.

Dr. Petracek entered the pod where I was waiting after hearing the results of my arteriogram. It was confirmed; I had a tear in my aorta and would definitely need immediate surgery. He, having just finished the heated discussion, was somewhat red-faced, immediately ordering everyone out of my room—the film crew, the cameras—only a couple of my friends were allowed to remain.

I learned early in life to smile in the face of adversity, so I greeted him with a smile despite what I'd just heard in their *discussion* next door. I have wondered many times if he took my smile and positive attitude as maybe I wasn't taking my situation seriously, so he launched into my diagnosis and concerns with the same intensity of his last discussion moments before and he informed me of all that could go wrong. While he was speaking—facing my bed with the door to his back—I saw the long boom with the attached microphone enter the room far over his head to capture his words while the camera was fixed on us outside the door. In a quick glance, I saw Barbara Kopple press her index finger over her lips to signal me not to give that overhead mic away. I had to suppress a smile for fear he would see the mic and demand them out. Then he began telling me how he would take an aorta with an aortic sleeve from a cadaver—frozen and preserved for such a time as this. He would actually choose two aortic valves and sleeves from six or seven donors. Then prepare two of those just in case one failed or ripped. It sounded futuristic. In the end, I would need an aortic valve and four inches of aorta grafted.

The aorta is made up of three layers of tissue; the tunica intima, tunica media, and tunica adventitia. A weakness or a nick forms on the inside layer, caused over time by trauma, disease, tissue disease, etc., for reasons unknown. Then a little plaque of calcium gets in that nick and when the blood hits it, it separates. This dissects the intima and media. All the nerves located there caused my extreme pain and temporary paralysis in the lake in Holland, when it occurred. The nerve endings transmit the pain as it tears. That pain is felt in the back and left shoulder as it goes down the descending aorta towards the stomach, as the nerve endings are torn. If the top layer, the tunica adventitia, tears, you bleed out very quickly. Thankfully, my top layer did not tear despite my activities after the original trauma, including 7 airline flights, bike riding and exercise, all while on prescription blood thinners!

Repairing the dissection can stop blood flow even during or after the surgery. All the blood vessels branch off of the aorta, and that can cause strokes, paralysis, blindness, and death of your bowels and intestines. It was explained to me recently that when my aorta dissected, that caused an immediate drop in blood pressure, which probably caused my paralysis in the water. As I floated in the water, unable to move my limbs, over time the blood pressure increased, and the paralysis lessened allowing me to regain feeling, eventually to climb out of the water and onto the boat.

My risk at the time was very high. Adding to that risk was the physician in Holland only ordered an EKG, which would not show the dissection. According to Dr. Petracek, putting me on a bicycle treadmill before doing a CT scan or MRI was very dangerous.

Though the cardiologist in Hungary could see the tear during the echocardiogram, and in Nashville by way of the arteriogram, they had no way of knowing the actual size of the tear. Once Dr. Petracek opened my chest, he could actually see evidence of the original tear, some healing, then more tearing, and healing. This occurred over the weeks that I continued life as usual after the Dutch hospital release. A dissection has huge risks on any level, but once the surgeon and his team were inside my chest and saw the size and length of the tear, the operation became even more serious. He said, "There was scar tissue, and the outer layer of tissue was very thin. I was surprised it had not ruptured. But things happen for a reason."

He said if I had been diagnosed correctly in that first emergency room, it would have meant immediate surgery in Holland. However, rather than a homograft, I would have received a mechanical valve or a pig-tissue valve and a Gore-Tex sleeve. There were organ banks in Europe, but there were few, if any, tissue banks in 1997. Whether in Holland or in Hungary, the outcome could have been much different. The risks would have been much higher with a mechanical valve and Gore-Tex sleeve, due to more bleeding, transfusions, and the possibility of rejecting the replacement parts.

The homograft was not in vogue 25 years ago; however, Dr. Petracek thought I would have better longevity, given my age of 45, by using a homograft. He said choosing the right size was based on blood type, actual size of the graft, and the size of my aorta.

I recently sat down with Michael Petracek at his home just outside of Nashville. We visited for more than three hours. He remembered my surgery well and was so kind to allow me to ask lots of questions that I had been pondering for many years. I was not surprised at all to hear his philosophy in all of his years of surgery and patient care. He told me that he treated every one of his patients like family, and they are still his family. He said that doing his best was how he got through the hard times, even the loss of a patient. He got the best people around him, the best referring doctors, the best equipment, and the best hardware, or in my case, the best homograft. He also believed the outcome was predetermined by God. Michael Petracek told me that day that he had always thought, "How can someone trust their life to someone they do not know? If they put that trust in you, you had better do every possible thing for them, or you have betrayed them."

He went on to say, "Being a physician is like being part of the patient's family. Patients want to be touched, they want to talk, they want to ask questions." He said he always touched his patients, which enhanced his ability to sense their anxiety level. "You want a patient to trust you; that comes partly from touch, and trust is important for a positive outcome." I do remember his hand upon my shoulder when he talked to me 25 years ago!

The day I met Petracek back in 1997, I was overall at peace, because I knew in my heart that God had not brought me this far, over 9 weeks, multiple flights and countries, to leave me now. I had full confidence I would come through the surgery with flying colors and live more life. Though confident I would make it, there were still some pretty dark hours ahead.

I was admitted to the hospital, and the surgery was planned for the next morning. I was only allowed up for bathroom visits and nothing else. That afternoon word spread that I was scheduled for a very big surgery the next morning. That evening, family and friends started arriving to see me, with lots of love and laughter, hugs and prayers. All of this social time, despite having lights, cameras, and action… a full film crew in my room.

Sometime mid evening, the cardiologist, Dr. Mark Glazer, visited me on his rounds and found the hallway and my room full of people laughing and talking—just hanging out. He made his way to my bed and nicely scolded me. He said, with a smile, that I needed to clear the room and get some rest. I reminded him that

I had just returned from a long stint overseas, and had not seen friends and family for a long time. He reminded me that I was having serious open-heart surgery early in the morning. Then I did what he asked, and before the group left, they surrounded me to pray. Special times with special people.

Early the next morning I awoke for surgery prep. After that extreme exfoliating process was over, I was happy to see friends back again to pray for me and pray for God's continued protection. They also prayed for my surgeon, and continued to pray as other friends came in and out of the waiting room throughout the 7 hour procedure.

Having had the surgery filmed, some months afterward I asked for, and was granted permission, to watch the surgery. Saint Thomas allowed me to watch on the condition that I was with the Director of Patient Relations, Cathy Osteen. Watching the video, I heard two very important statements: After opening my chest, Dr. Petracek said that the bubble of tissue which held my aorta together was as thin as tissue paper. He also said, "The Lord must surely have his hand on this young man. This rip is huge, and I can't believe he survived it."

Petracek had predicted the strong possibility of a couple of blood transfusions either during or after the surgery. Though we made it through the surgery without a transfusion there were some tense moments late in the night concerning my blood pressure. The attending nurse called the surgeon at home and he instructed them to give me a bit more time in hopes that my blood pressure would come back up on its own; if it did not, then he would approve the transfusion. Thankfully, it came back up on its own and I credit that to God's grace, His angels charged to watch over me, and the prayers of many both at home and abroad.

FEBRUARY 23, 1998

AdvertisingAge

Hospital spots dose reality with restraint

[BOB GARFIELD'S AD REVIEW]

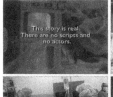

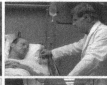

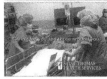

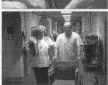

"T his story is real," reads the super that opens each of six serialized spots for St. Thomas Health Services in Nashville. "There are no scripts and no actors."

Rather, we're witness to a real-life crisis. Oscar-winning documentarian Barbara Kopple follows the case of 46-year-old Randy Morgan, who presents with a diseased aorta and undergoes high-risk surgery to repair it.

"This is not a simple, straightforward problem," we see the surgeon inform him. "This is much more severe than we thought it was...he has a high risk of dying from the complications."

A 20%-30% risk, he's told. It's terrifying, but Kopple and Nashville agency Endres Eng Wilson don't milk the melodrama, delivering instead subtle human moments of breathtaking poignancy.

"I want to see my brothers," Morgan announces upon hearing the prognosis. And then, trying to cheerfully confront the worst case: "If this is it, I've had a good time, you know."

Who needs a script with reality like that?

We see a silent prayer. When the surgeons open him up, we see their stunned reaction to the torn aorta that by rights should have killed him. And, of course, in the end we see Morgan walk out of the hospital, all fixed up.

There's the rub. Had the outcome been different, it wouldn't be on TV. If Morgan had died in surgery, or had a stroke in the recovery room, the film wouldn't even have been developed.

As genuine and moving as this story is, it is also, like previous "documercials," built upon underlying deception: the failure to acknowledge that the story's outcome—unlike the patient's, unlike any St. Thomas patient's—is a foregone conclusion.

In that sense, there's a certain Hollywood-thriller quality to it. Just as we knew Sandra Bullock wasn't going to blow up on the bus in "Speed," we know this guy isn't going to die. ("That, after all, would send the wrong brand message. The "Caring for You and Those Around You" tagline may be lame, but it's better than "St. Thomas. Hey, Nobody Bats 1,000").

That we willingly suspend uncertainty about whether the patient will live allows the drama to survive, but what about truth? If a documentary implies documenting what happens, come what may, isn't there something dishonest when the come-what-may is removed from the equation?

The answer is yes. When Eastern Airlines used this technique in its last-ditch effort to win consume sympathy, its self-serving selectivity of the footage underlined its propagandisti falsity. When e.p.t. filmed "real people" reading their pregnancy results, it screamed of tabloid-TV exploitiveness.

What distinguishes this campaign—and redeems it—is its understatement and restraint.

To the credit of the advertiser and its agency, the selective truth is an unadorned truth. There is no suggestion, for instance, that St. Thomas somehow takes the fear out of health crises or gives you better odds against death. Indeed, it rather chillingly documents how lucky this guy was to make it to surgery, much less through it.

And it communicates the notion of care not by showing pillow-fluffing nurses or heroic surgeons in hand-to-scythe battle with the Grim Reaper, but by showing competent professionals soberly going about their business.

Their brutal candor is, paradoxically, confidence-inspiring—which is precisely what the campaign intends. This may not be true documentary, but it is a remarkable document nonetheless. ☐

St. Thomas Health Services: *Endres Eng Wilson, Nashville, Tenn.*
Ad Review rating ★ ★ ★ ½

49

I had not walked into Saint Thomas Hospital that day planning on being in a real life docu-drama. I was there because I fought to get home to Nashville from Europe. I needed the support and touch of family and friends. Being filmed and in 6 commercials was never in my wildest dreams when getting on the plane in Budapest. Yet, God had a story for me to tell, and He kept me alive to tell it through these commercials, because nearly 18% of those who suffer an aortic dissection die before arriving at the hospital and 21% die within 24 hours if they do not have surgery.

So I was a walking miracle, soon to become an advertising sensation that would land my face on the cover of *Ad Age* and other magazines, newsprint, as well as television commercials. Is this what I really wanted? Lights, cameras, and crew capturing my most vulnerable moments, then airing them on television? I wasn't sure, but the commercials became a catalyst of hope.

The Bread Truck with Randy Travis and Australia with the Mandrells

Back in Nashville, after my Dallas stint, the Peavys offered me the opportunity to open an Alaman's Mexican Restaurant in Nashville. After long conversations and looking around for some higher end properties, I accepted the opportunity. A beautiful old house was found on the corner of Louise Avenue and State Street near West End and Vanderbilt University. The house had been a restaurant before, so the kitchen was already setup somewhat in the basement of this grand old place. Architecturally, it lent itself well to an upscale Mexican villa. Above the basement kitchen there were two main floors, plus an attic office. Four flights of steps—good thing that I was only 28 years old.

After a few months of minor renovations and purchases, we were ready for opening night. I hosted two free invitation-only nights. This gave the staff the chance to have a dress rehearsal before the public opening the following week. I remember enjoying so many of my friends on those two evenings.

We had almost immediate success. At that time, there was only one other Mexican restaurant that was not a chain. It was on the southeast side, and though it had been there for years, it was not a great part of town at that time. Elliston Place, however, was "the" place to be, with the Exit Inn and a new TGI Fridays on the next block. Due to my music business relationships and connections, we hosted a few Album Release Parties for the record label companies like RCA and SONY Music on Nashville's nearby Music Row. A number of country music bands would come for dinner before boarding their tour busses. Some would even get picked up at the restaurant to go on tour. I remember some of the Charlie Daniels band loved Alaman's.

Unfortunately, I was not ready for success at this point in my life, and the pressures of the restaurant got to me. The long days, from dawn till the wee hours of the next, eventually wore me down. It has been said that one is truly married to a restaurant. It was more than full-time, and I was not doing well. At first, I would have a Happy Hour drink in the afternoon as we prepared for the evening crowd, then two drinks… it soon developed into a "keep'm comin' bartender" until we closed around 2:00am. I began to move my personal happy hour up earlier and earlier, and it wasn't long before I was having a drink before we were open for the lunch crowd. Needless to say I was maintaining a constant buzz drinking from morning until closing—every day. I was practically living at the restaurant.

At this time, my wife was traveling and singing with Jim Ed Brown. She was *on the road* quite often for days at a time and at The Opry on the weekends when they were in town. I remember one evening she came to the restaurant and told me she wanted a divorce. I think I knew it was coming. Still, I was surprised. A lot happened in those next days and weeks following, but I made the decision to leave the restaurant and attempt to save my marriage.

After resigning and negotiating my departure from Alaman's, my previous boss and friend, Bill, and I talked through opening a paint and wallpaper store in Hendersonville, TN, just northeast of Nashville. A lot of country music artists, pickers and singers, lived in this town next to Old Hickory Lake, and I was familiar with the area. Within a few months we were up and running with a Home

Decorating Center. It was a nice location backing up to the lake. Hendersonville was growing with lots of new construction and renovations. There was only one other paint and wallpaper store in the community at the time. So I started decorating again at the Home Center.

Because of friendships and our connections at the Grand Ole Opry, a number of opportunities opened up for me to provide decorating services for notables like Mr. Roy Acuff, Sharon and Ricky Skaggs, and The Nashville Network executive and Hee Haw Television directors, Anne and Bob Boatman.

One of my most noteworthy decorating jobs was when Opryland USA built a house for Roy Acuff, the King of Country Music. WSM and the top brass at Opryland began to give some thought to an aging Mr. Acuff who had recently lost his wife Mildred. They had a beautiful old home on the Inglewood side of the Cumberland River, overlooking what was then Opryland USA. Though just across the river, it took 15 to 20 minutes to drive each way. Opryland decided they would build him a residence on the property beside The Opry House. Upon completion, Mr. Acuff sold his Moss Rose home and moved into the Opryland House, which was named the Acuff Museum.

Mr. Acuff worked closely with my friend Debbie Logue, and he mentioned to her that he needed help with some decor decisions in the new house. Debbie offered my help and the rest is history. I went to his house and helped Mr. Roy decide what he would take to the new house and I made drawings of the window treatments. He wanted that same traditional look in the new house that he and Mildred had enjoyed in their beautiful old white-columned house on the bluff of the river.

The decorating job for Mr. Acuff led into working for Anne and Bob Boatman in their home on Winding Way in Inglewood, and later a new home on the historic Hazel Path Mansion grounds in Hendersonville. This also led to a summer part-time renovation of their cabin cruiser boat docked on Old Hickory Lake. I enjoyed many afternoons with Anne and Bob on the lake. Bob was the director of the popular country television show *Hee Haw*, and he had been lighting consultant to four U.S. Presidents before moving to Nashville, and marrying Anne. I spent a lot of time with Bob and Anne in design work and socially. Bob called me the *Don Rickles of Country Music* because of my sarcasm and one liners. We enjoyed many laughs together. Sadly he was killed in an apparent accident in his home in Hendersonville during the summer of 1989, and Anne passed in 2019 after a long battle with Alzheimer's.

In the early 80s my wife was still singing with Jim Ed Brown and we were still spending a lot of time on the weekends at The Grand Ole Opry. I had seen Sharon and Ricky Skaggs backstage at The Opry numerous times. Soon after we opened the decorating business, they purchased a house in Hendersonville. Since I had worked on the interior design for the previous owners, Sharon came by our store one day and asked if I would help her redo a guest room into a baby nursery. I helped her pick out wallpaper and paint for the nursery renovations and was actually there at the house putting the finishes touches on the nursery when Sharon went into labor. Molly Skaggs was born later that night or early the next morning. Molly is a worship leader today and very much a talent in her own right—how could she miss?

The decorating store was successful but as with all new businesses, it takes time to pay off the original investment of stock and opening costs. In addition, my business partner developed cancer, and, due to treatments, was often unable to work. He was diagnosed with a fast-growing form of cancer and after a couple of years, the strain of the center became too much. It was decided that we would have to close and file for bankruptcy. That was very difficult for us all, those of us who worked there and our investors. We all lost, but my partner and I were forced into personal bankruptcy as well. That was very difficult for me in that it brought back those old feelings that my father had said, "You will never amount to anything." I thought about that constantly in that period. I had failed... he was right.

After we closed the decorating center, my wife and I moved back into Green Hills and once again lived with our college friends, Doug and Marky. They lived in the old Goodpasture home on Caldwell Lane in Oak Hill. It was a big old house and we had all lived together before, so it felt like coming home. One afternoon a friend called to tell me that Louise Mandrell was looking for two blonde female backup singers for her new show. Louise was the brunette of the three Mandrell sisters, so it made sense that she wanted blondes. I asked my friend that day if she would consider a married couple... one blonde girl and her high-tenor husband, who was blondish, well, after some 'Sun-In'.

We auditioned and were asked to do a show with Louise. We did a few shows together, and I enjoyed singing with Louise and her band, but I needed steady work. Louise hired Dianne, and I took a position with the Country Music Association (CMA).

At CMA, I began answering the phone and overseeing the reception area. Soon however, there was an opening in the planning department assisting the notorious Helen Farmer who oversaw the planning and execution of the annual CMA Awards and Fan Fair.

Fan Fair began in 1972 at Nashville's Municipal Auditorium in downtown Nashville. By the early 80s it had outgrown that venue and moved to south Nashville at the Tennessee State Fairgrounds. There were concerts day and night at the Nashville Speedway, with dual stages set right on the front stretch of the track. Artists' booths, where fans could meet the stars, get a photo and autographs, were in the barns and buildings surrounding the track.

In 2001, CMA moved the festival back downtown with outdoor stages on Broadway and Riverfront Park which allowed the guests to not only take in the festival events, but peruse the honky tonks and clubs that have become so popular. In 2004, Fan Fair became CMA Fest.

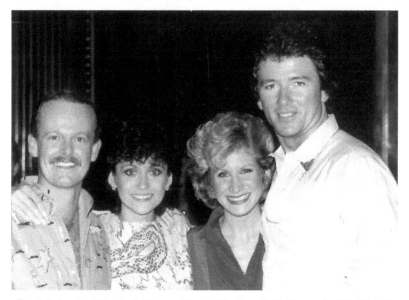

Randall, Louise Mandrell, Dianne, Patrick Duffy at R.C. Bannon's 40th Birthday party, Hermitage Hotel, Nashville

I had the pleasure of coordinating and playing host to many artists' fan clubs and their fans. Something like 25,000 people per day attended Fan Fair in the mid 80s and honestly, it was a blast! I enjoyed meeting some notables I had seen on television and listened to on the radio as a teenager. Not only did Fan Fair attract country artists, there were a number of pop artists who were *crossing over* at that time like the Nitty Gritty Dirt Band.

I had a number of amazing experiences, like having lunch with my friend Debbie, Grand Ole Opry Manager Hal Durham, and pop icon, American Bandstand personality, Dick Clark. The 70s and 80s were major growth years for country music and its national and international popularity. Music groups that had been pop groups came to Nashville, and it seemed that country music engulfed pop music as rock music took its own direction.

I also connected with two of my early Christian influencers that I knew from The Opry. Sharon White, of The Whites, and Ricky Skaggs. They were always kind to everyone, and I knew they were devoted Christians, and though I was not, I knew enough to appear as a Christian. A few years later, Ricky and Sharon gave me a book which I still have today. *The Search for Significance* by Robert McGee. They gave it to me as a gift before I moved to Nigeria the summer of 1989. That book really helped me get through some challenging days during my time in West Africa.

Recently, September of 2019, I saw Ricky and Sharon at Community Church of Hendersonville. Ricky performed special music in the service that morning and I was delighted to see them along with Sharon's dad, Buck White. The Whites, Grand Ole Opry members since '84, have been called "the first family of country music".

While working at CMA I also enjoyed being involved in the planning and execution of the CMA Awards show and all that this entailed. Music business executives were involved in the planning by serving on committees, and we hosted numerous meetings to plan every aspect of the show. I was fortunate to meet and build relationships with a number of music row executives during that time. One of those was American Society of Composers, Authors and Publishers executive Connie Bradley. Connie had mentioned privately that she wanted to hire me to work at ASCAP, but did not have any positions open at that time but would call when she did.

My two years at CMA were truly unforgettable as I enjoyed so many aspects of the awards shows and Fan Fair but the pay was low and I wanted more. I admit, I did not know what that *more* was going to be, but I figured something would come along soon enough. I resigned from the CMA early in 1985.

Randy Travis had signed with Warner Brothers and was getting a lot of airplay by spring of 1985. One evening I was talking with Randy and his manager, Lib Hatcher, and they asked if I wanted to help them on the road for a bit. The band traveled in the infamous "Bread Truck," and I drove Randy and Lib in their private customized van. I drove, helped sell his merchandise, and sang backup adding some high harmonies. The funny thing is that I also acted as his bodyguard, bringing him through the crowds to the stage at the venues. Randy and I are about the same height, but Randy was an avid weightlifter and exerciser, so it is more than comical that I had him by the arm pushing our way through excited fans who wanted to stop him, speak to him, hug him, you name it. Thankfully I was able to get him to the stage and was never challenged beyond what I could push through or push him through.

I worked with Randy for his first three singles, "1982," "On the Other Hand," "Diggin' Up Bones." I left just after the release of "I'm Gonna Love You Forever." I always enjoyed singing with Randy. His voice was low and consistent; singing harmony with him was easy because of that consistency. As a high tenor, I sang almost an octave apart from Randy. He used to say of me, "That boy sings higher than a dog whistle." But the road life was not for me. It was tiring and certainly not glamorous. For that enjoyable hour on stage, singing at Gilley's, Billy Bob's in Fort Worth or any number of country 2-step clubs between Austin and New Orleans, there were 23 hours in the day that were not so glamorous.

Randy and Lib loved the restaurant chain Cracker Barrel Old Country Stores. We ate at Cracker Barrel restaurants from

Tennessee to Texas and back again. Then there was the driving through the night to the next gig, the next city, the next motel to get cleaned up, and then off to the club for soundcheck, only to have it start all over again. So life on the road was not the life for me. We did, however, have some good laughs, and it was easy to get caught up in the energy of Randy's emerging career.

The guys in the band were fun. Rocky Thacker was playing bass, Drew Sexton was on the piano, and Randy Hardison was the drummer. Hardison was always ready for a laugh, and he and Rocky were usually the instigators of the fun. One weekend we were in Dallas, Texas to do a joint concert downtown with Tanya Tucker and The Osmonds. That afternoon I went with Randy and Lib to a reception that the Dallas mayor was hosting. When I returned to get ready for the concert, I found my hair brush had been remodeled and all the teeth had been pulled out, except for maybe seven. Funny thing is—it still worked. I was still able to comb my hair, which made the guys laugh even louder when I told them. There were good times. Randy and Lib were warm and enjoying this new era. It was literally the answer to their prayers and dreams. It was sweet to see Randy's singles climbing in the charts.

Some years later, while in Europe, one evening streaming what American programming I could find, I ran across a television show that my dad would have called a "whodunnit." I was watching an episode of *48 Hours*, a true-crime series, about a Nashville murder. Something sounded familiar about this man who was found beaten and later died. As I sat there and watched, it became clear to me that I knew this guy. It was Randy Hardison, the drummer with Randy Travis, and our Nashville Palace days. He had been murdered in Nashville, and it was later reported that maybe he was having an affair with a man's wife. What a waste. Randy was a super talented guy, writing songs for Lee Ann Womack, Garth Brooks and Darryl Worley.

After that spring on the road with Randy Travis, Connie Bradley contacted me and I was hired for a position at ASCAP. My original position was completing the paperwork for songwriters to join and also setting up publishing companies for songwriters and publishers. ASCAP is a membership organization so approval is required of songwriters and publishing companies.

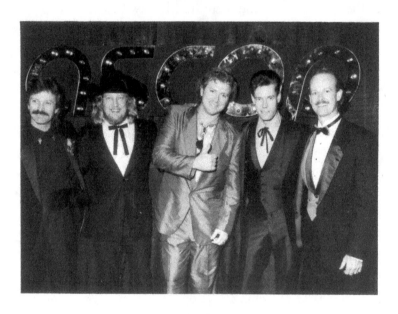

Jeff Hanna, John Anderson, T Graham Brown, Randy Travis, Randall Morgan
Photo Credit: 1998 by Don Putnam

It was during my time at ASCAP that my marriage took its final turn. Spring of '87 my wife and I went to Australia with the Mandrell sisters for a television taping in the world class Sydney Opera House. *Australia Salutes Country Music* or was it *Country Music Salutes Australia*? I can't really remember. The journey was long but enjoyable on many levels, yet there was an underlying sadness also. My wife and I had been separated for some time by that point, and maybe we thought that this time away would breathe new life, new hope into our marriage.

Being raised in *the church*, there were a lot of Do's and Don'ts. Often, I felt the Don'ts outweighed the Do's, but that could have just been my perception. One thing I understood from my religious upbringing was the big Don't of divorce. I had witnessed the devastation of divorce in my extended family and had heard the whispers of divorce in my church congregation once or twice. I knew it caused lots of pain, and even though I'd heard it was not the unforgivable sin, it sure seemed pretty unforgivable to me.

I had said numerous times that I did not want a divorce. Yet, in the quiet of my heart, I knew the marriage was over and possibly should never have been. This is my story, not hers, so I can only speak for me when I say that I was ill-prepared for marriage.

Summer and Autumn of '87 found me partying a lot. I was drinking and doing occasional recreational drugs, trying to mask my shame and maybe appearing not to care, yet I cared deeply. I just did not know how to communicate the pain, or to whom to communicate. When I married, there was never a question in my mind, I was marrying for keeps—*till death do us part*. So when I knew that my marriage was over, I was depressed. I felt like the loser my dad said I would be.

— 12 —

My Bloody Mary Morning

In my childhood, both of my parents had struggled with depression, and I saw firsthand the hopelessness they felt. Now, here I was in my mid 30s and feeling the same. I was truly fighting hopelessness.

Due to the fact that I was extremely social, my hopelessness was masked almost entirely by an *I don't care* attitude. I had learned the art of masking early in life to decrease the pain of shame. A number of my friends and people I worked with in the music business liked to hang out at the local bars. So drinking was really a norm for us. After work, it was off to Maude's Courtyard, Tavern on The Row, Third Coast, or any number of local hangouts for Happy Hour. The time I spent drinking and laughing allowed me to avoid my real feelings for at least a few hours. Then there was the *last call for alcohol* and the drive home. I can not tell you how many times I drove home well above the alcohol limit. One evening, I had only driven a block or so when the blue lights of a police cruiser approached from behind. My heart thumped wildly as he ask me for my car papers. After a quick check, he cautioned me to slow down and did not even mention a breathalyzer. He gave me back my license, with a warning to "head home" and drive safely. A sane person would have vowed at that moment to never let this happen again. Sadly, it would take more than this one incident to shake me from the depth of my hopelessness. As I started the car and pulled away I kind of sped off with a bit of tail spray of gravel.

Back on the road, I had not even gone two blocks when again, I was looking at the blue lights flashing in my rearview mirror. This officer had noticed my tail spray of gravel from the previous stop, and I guess it looked as if I was angry or simply *out of control*. Believe it or not, this officer also gave me only a warning and sent me on my way, encouraging me to get home and rest. This officer actually said to me, "I can tell you have been drinking." Still he let me go with only a warning. Surely, this was the wakeup call I needed! Two stops within a 15-minute period. Both officers letting me go with only a warning. You'd think I'd stop drinking and driving, but nope, not me. I quickly took it for granted and the next week I was back to my old ways of drinking and driving. Back to my old ways of trying to fill this horrible void—this black hole in my soul that could not be filled with *drugs, sex and rock and roll*, or country music, as it were.

I have often thought that we spend our childhood and young adult years slapping band-aids on our hurts, both physically and emotionally. Life is full and busy, and this helps us defer the pain. We cover the cut, the sore, the damaged skin or feelings with something that numbs the pain, and then we move on quickly to the *next thing*, the *next laugh*, the *next opportunity*, the *next drink*, the *next drug*. We spend years doing the coverup. When we enter our 40's—some older and some younger—we realize that the adhesive no longer holds the band-aids on, and they drop off. The pains of our past are indeed still there and still hurt. So what do we do? We try and stick them back on or add new ones—new drugs, new drinks, new partying. That was what I did, I partied more. Then shame and guilt overpowered me again. Partying can only temporarily mask the pain. Sadness and emotional pain can wait out the party, only to resurface, and then the hopelessness is even greater. We can't run from ourselves. Believe me, I tried.

During this season, one of my responsibilities at the office was to finalize the paperwork for new publishing companies. My experience with most applicants was very positive and I enjoyed working with many songwriters and music publishers.

One of the applicants that I worked with during that season was Integrity Hosanna Music, a Christian music organization in Mobile, Alabama. We worked together for a number of weeks reserving the name of the publishing company and completing the necessary documents. They were great to work with and we soon finalized their membership with ASCAP.

To show their appreciation for my work, they sent me their complete library of cassette tapes, which were in the dozens at that time. It was a very thoughtful gift, but I remember thinking, "What am I going to do with these?" By this time, I had not attended church in years. So to hear these tapes of worship songs with full instrumentation felt confusing. On one hand I enjoyed the sound, but I felt conflicted, based on my religious childhood of non-instrumental music in church. So I took the nicely packaged cassettes home and put them on a shelf in my music closet.

Life went on, partying continued. As those aforementioned band-aids continued to fall off, the realization of my failures consumed more and more of my thoughts, and my unhappiness continued to grow. With the growth of unhappiness came the realization of fear in my life. My fear was that I had failed, not only *had* failed, but was truly a *failure*. My father was correct: "I would never amount to anything." I internalized this message and reinforced it at the bottom of every glass. *Failure!*

In late autumn of that year, the darkness of winter evenings set in earlier and earlier, mirroring my unhappiness… moving toward despair. The only joy was that the Christmas season was approaching and I have always loved Christmas. But even Christmas could be a bitter sweet time for me. As a child, it was a magical time in my heart, and yet it became the saddest time after my mother was diagnosed with cancer. My father reminded me every year that *this will probably be your mother's last Christmas*. I had heard that since I was 12, and throughout my teen years, until I was out of my parent's home and into college. So Christmas was not the easiest time for me.

As I moved through the holiday season with all of its activities, I was able to keep my party face on. At that time, the Music Row area of Nashville was very much a community with all the major record label offices, publishers, recording studios within walking distance of ASCAP, BMI, and CMA. The Music Row community welcomed any reason to party and it was full-on ready from Christmas, through summer Fan Fair, autumn's CMA week, ASCAP, BMI and SESAC Awards banquets, the Harlan Howard Birthday Bash street party, and back to the next Christmas. One year we created a Music Row Halloween parade and I borrowed a friend's MG T and drove my friend Suzanne Lee around posing as the *1954 ASCAP Pumpkin Queen*. (Sorry about that clutch, Kirk and Rhonda.)

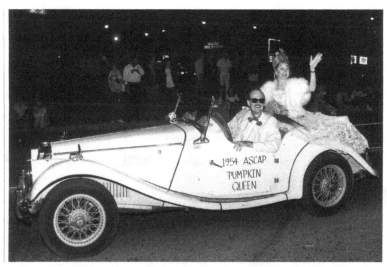

By December '87, I was reaching the end of my ability to comfort myself with partying and drinking. I was miserable. I was sad and hopeless. In the evenings after drinking, I would return to my condominium and dig out those Integrity Hosanna cassette tapes and listen to the songs. Some of the earlier releases were "Give Thanks (with a grateful heart)", "Mighty God," "Lord of All," the list is too lengthy to write. As I would listen to these songs, my heart was strangely consoled. Yet, I could not allow myself to believe that even if there was a God, he cared about me, or wanted to have a relationship with me. I felt alone.

Within the religious context of my childhood, I knew how to jump through the hoops of what I thought Christianity required. I was even baptized twice in my teens. The first time was the summer of my 13th year when I stepped out into the church aisle and walked to the front while the congregation sang "Just as I Am." I am sorry to say that I really did not go forward for baptism that day because of my sincere belief. I walked that aisle because my father had a well-intentioned talk with me about our upcoming drive from Tennessee to Oklahoma. The possibility of being killed in an accident and going straight to Hell, because I was not baptized, was my motivation. I wanted to believe in God. I looked for God and prayed to God, but never really felt anything. I just settled into religious life, trying to be good. For me… that seemed difficult.

One Friday evening, just after the new year, January of 1988, I left work at ASCAP and headed off to one of my hangouts with music business friends. We shared a bottle or three of wine and probably some appetizers, but soon it was time for me to go home. I had drunk way too much and, as usual lied to myself that I was okay to drive, so I did, though I would not remember that drive the next morning.

The following morning was Saturday, and I awoke very sick. My head was pounding. I felt nauseated, so I just lay there listening to my heartbeat in my temples. This was certainly not my first hangover, so I knew what I needed to do, I knew the drill. But as I lay there in my bed summoning the strength to stand, I wondered about the evening before. Where was I, and how did I get home? Unable to fully reconstruct the evening, I finally threw my legs off the side of the bed and stood up, swaying a bit from side to side and swallowing back the nausea, knowing that I was still intoxicated. I knew that I needed a drink, a bit of "hair of the dog (that bit you)" as they say. It adds some alcohol back into your system to numb the effects of the dehydration, which was the cause of the headache and the nausea. On my way to the kitchen I stopped at my living room window to look out. My car was there. I had driven home drunk, blind drunk this time. I had no memory of that journey. That created such fear in me. I can still remember the sinking feeling to this day. What if? What if I had wrecked the car? What if I had killed someone on the road? All of these put such fear into me. The *what ifs* of life!

I turned on my stereo and one of the Integrity Hosanna tapes began a worship song. I walked into the kitchen and began making my drink, a Bloody Mary, which is tomato juice and vodka with a healthy splash of Tabasco hot sauce, a good squirt of lemon or lime, salt and pepper and voila, a soothing balm of alcohol that would hopefully help to reduce the sickness that I was feeling. As I returned to the living room, with drink in hand, the reality of my unhappiness came upon me with such force that I was barely able to place the drink on my sofa table before the tears began to run down my cheeks. At that moment, I knew I could not continue life as I knew it, as I had been living it. I was miserable, I was lost, and the worst was that I was without hope. As I stood there in my living room, feeling hopeless, I looked up and said, "If there is a God, heal me or kill me, because I do not want to live like this anymore." With that poor excuse of a prayer, God reached down in His mercy and touched me. I collapsed onto the floor and began to weep. I am not talking about little eye-watering tears, but gut-wrenching emotion. Years of pain and confusion, self-hatred, inadequacies covered by my humor, loss and grief of what could have been, maybe what should have been, came out in those tears.

I am being completely honest when I say that I had never encountered God before that moment. All the religion in which I had been raised, did not prepare me for encountering the God of the Universe, the Creator, God, who knit me together in my mother's womb. As I cried the pain out, God was so gracious to allow His comfort to console my heart. After crying for what felt like hours, I began to feel peace. Then joy, true joy was taking over my heart and my mind, and I began to smile and then to laugh. After a time of basking in that joy and resting in the truth of knowing, for the first time, that there is a God, and I am His... feeling His love... my Father's Love. Wow!

After hours on the floor of my home, I got on my feet and picked up that watered-down Bloody Mary that had puddled, as iced drinks do, and as I wiped the table clean, it occurred to me that I was completely sober and without any sign of a hangover. I had not even taken a sip from that drink, yet my headache and nausea were gone. I was healed! What? I felt great. Not only did I feel great in my head and stomach, but I felt happy in my heart. For the first time in my life, I was content and at peace.

That was an amazing day and it completely changed my life. Early the next morning, I read the biblical account of Saul of Tarsus encountering Jesus on the road to Damascus in Acts 9. That Saturday in January of 1988 was my Damascus Road encounter.

— 13 —

I Think We Should Pull The Plug

I do not know if I would have made the same decision to be in the Saint Thomas Hospital commercials if I had been given a week, or even a day, to mull it over. The way it went down, I believe, was ordained by God. So being a sudden decision made it easier, and maybe I welcomed the distraction more than the idea of being filmed. Looking back, it is funny to think that these commercials were being planned for months prior to that week when I appeared at the hospital, even while I struggled for life in a Dutch lake—so far from home. It is amazing when you sit back and think about the timing of everything that happened. Just think of all the things that had to line up for me to be in those commercials. A whole filming crew was there, not for me, but—in the end—there for me. Maybe I had the dramatic flair they desired, which basically meant I talked and interacted. I smiled. I had a community of friends willing to be extras. I believe God had ordained this moment.

Kevin Endres of Endres Wilson Ad Agency, who had come up with the idea of a commercial docu-drama, said to me recently that there was even a moment when he was ready to stop the project. Once he heard the actual diagnosis and possible prognosis from Petracek, he walked outside of the hospital and called his business partner and said, "I think we should pull the plug and cut our losses." His partner talked him off the ledge. He went back in and filming was already underway. This is when Barbara Kopple turned to him and said, "This is great, possibly the best thing I have ever filmed."

Kevin also told me, during our recent chat over a cup of coffee, though I had the worst diagnosis, the worst chances of even getting back home, the worst chances for recovery, I got the best. The best care with the full weight of the hospital on my case, with the best doctors, nurses, technicians. The best materials with the homograph aortic valve, plus inches of aortic sleeve, large enough to graft into my damaged tissue. Ultimately the best with God's story to be told, so that I would give Him the glory. He takes the worst and gives the best.

I am not sure what my surgery would have been like without the filming of the commercials. They say a doctor and patient enter into a partnership, facing obstacles together. In my case there were even more partners with the director, film crew, hospital staff, family, friends and prayer partners worldwide who were invested in the success of the surgery.

Autumn of 2021, I spent a few hours with Dr. Petracek at his home. I had not seen him since my follow-up visits in the weeks following the surgery. He has retired from surgery but still lectures at Vanderbilt University Medical Center. He looked genuinely happy to see me, and to see me doing so well. It was good for me to see him, and to have the opportunity to ask some questions that I had been asking myself for almost 25 years.

One of my questions to Dr. Petracek was what was it like to be filmed for this seven-hour procedure. He said that being filmed was not out of the ordinary, in that he had been filmed many times for educational purposes. In my case, he admitted the cameras did add more tension in the room. Everyone was keenly aware that their movements and comments were being filmed. With that tension came anxiety, and the overall pressure went up considerably. An already precarious situation became even more so with cameras, lights and crew! But everyone hoped for a successful outcome.

A thread of hope ran through everyone involved, from my family and friends, the hospital staff, and the film crew that I had just met. Hope had brought me through the last weeks, and helped me get home to the States. This hope was in The Lord who had spared my life from drowning and helped me through everything the past nine weeks had thrown at me. Maybe even the film team going into surgery with me gave me the additional strength to engage the foe of fear. I could not let them down, which has been a motivator in my life. We were all invested here, we all had skin in the game, so to speak. Maybe it allowed us to exert a level of control over such a risky surgery. We believed we controlled the narrative, and this was the catalyst for hope. For inside this docu-drama, all of the hallmark emotions existed: fear, anxiety, obstacles, forecasting, glorious moments, tearful moments, hope, and victory. Everyone wanted the protagonist to win in the end. Knowing this created belief and expectancy, which are the main ingredients of hope. I had to survive and thrive for the story to be told. The lead character had to transform in the end. And my role in this drama was to keep hope alive, which is what being a missionary and a pastor is all about. We spread hope. So I knew how to do this.

I had often been hopeless as a child. When I met Jesus for the first time in 1988, I was filled with hope. Since then I have been on numerous ministry teams of hope. All the way from being in bands to being on the mission field organizing concerts and other ministries. So I was energized by everyone on the team as they believed in my success and the success of this ad campaign, which was nothing more than believing in the mission. And the mission was a good one, of course. But the story was better than what they had hoped for going into this project. The first explanation of the *why* of these ads was to hopefully create a response in men who are notoriously avoiders and procrastinators when it comes to seeing a heart doctor. Sounds boring, right? I think Barbara Kopple knew this. There was no real drama in the other narrative, then in walks a man with an aortic dissection who had a 30% chance of death and a risk of neurological damage. Now you have a drama!

Ad Age put our commercials like this: "And it communicates the notion of care not by showing pillow-fluffing nurses or heroic surgeons in hand-to-scythe battle with the Grim Reaper, but by showing competent professionals soberly going about their business. Their brutal candor is paradoxically, confidence-inspiring—which is precisely what the campaign intends." Even *Ad Age* picked up on what I felt going into surgery—that everyone was confident, inspired and hopeful.

I do not think Saint Thomas or Barbara Kopple would have described it this way the day I walked onto their set. They were trying to reduce fear and engage with procrastinators—the men and women who would ignore pains and put off seeing a doctor. They had no idea they were about to embark on *"brutal candor"* that inspired confidence. I am shocked that more hospitals have not used docu-dramas on social media. These days the platform is more economical than television. Plus, in an age where misinformation thrives, would not a real seeing-is-believing docu-drama bode well with the community? Most hospitals opt for commercials that make the staff and the hospital the heroes, which lacks confidence-inspiring moments. The patient is always the hero, not that I would say that back then. But most hospitals cannot help but make themselves the heroes, because they believe the narrative is about the hospital's image, not the transformation of the patient. Sure, they feature patients after they have recovered successfully, but we do not see the travail. And I still believe that the commercials Barbara Kopple directed captured the best indications of how a patient will be treated. Now, if I had died, maybe all of this would have been for naught. But this ad campaign supported the hope within me, and those around me. Kopple and her team became part of my family and friends. It exploited my natural tendency to be on a team, to be an integral part of a project. Was this really any different than going on stage with Randy Travis, Louise Mandrell, Jim Ed Brown or hearing my name announced on The Grand Ole Opry? I had been primed for this moment by everything that went before the surgery. I just needed to add a smile and maybe some charm. This team, this project, created additional hope that disintegrated the hopelessness that I felt sitting on that cold hospital bench in Budapest, trying to figure out my next move. Something propelled me along the streets of Budapest and onto those flights to get home to Nashville, where a docu-drama and a homograft were waiting. See the tapestry? Only God can work behind the scenes like this to give us the best possible chance of survival. I might have needed those commercials as much as they needed me. And maybe my doctors and the plethora of nurses and technicians needed them as well. Maybe it lifted their game. I am not sure, but I needed a team in those moments. I needed a narrative of hope.

A few years after my surgery and the commercials had received the awards, I was asked to be the keynote speaker for the Saint Thomas Nurses Appreciation banquet. I told the nurses that night that despite the glamour of the spotlight often shone on the doctors, it was the nurses who were often the ministers of hope. They were the human touch, the kind voice in the middle of the night when we are awakened by the noise of the machines, the breathing tube down our throats, the fear and disorientation; it was they who touched our lives with hope.

Shane J. Lopez puts it like this, in his book *Making Hope Happen*, "Simply by proximity, we can infect others with the mission and excitement of our pursuits. And being exposed to others' goals primes us to adopt them. Associate with people who share your goals, or the goals you want to be more salient, and you get an automatic boost in focus and motivation." This is called goal contagion, and I wish every hospital could create something that would cue hope the way those cameras cued hope within everyone associated with our commercials.

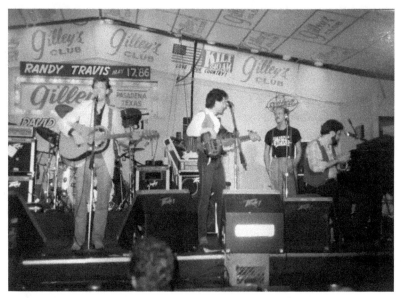

Randy Travis at Gilley's

Funny antidote: One evening while on the road with Randy Travis, during a concert at Mickey Gilley's nightclub in Pasadena, Texas, the audience was somewhat subdued, which was unusual. Randy was singing, "Send My Body Home on A Freight Train," and I started clapping to give the audience a cue to clap along as well. That was not an unusual thing for a backup singer to do, and the audience joined in immediately. After the show, Randy's manager Lib Hatcher came to me and said simply, "Morgan,"— she always called me Morgan because there was already Randy Travis and Randy Hardison in the band. So she said "Morgan, they came to see Randy Travis, not you, don't clap." So that was that. No clapping. I got the message. But she misinterpreted my intentions. I was not trying to steal the spotlight from Randy, I was trying to connect people, to Randy, the show, to each other. As I look back that seems to be a reoccurring theme in my life. I want to connect with people and see people connect with others.

I was not not looking for a spotlight in these St. Thomas commercials. In fact, if given some time to think about it, I might have declined. But, in that moment, I was motivated by being on the team, connecting with people and bringing others hope. As Oliver Wendall Holmes once said, "Beware how you take away hope from another person." I don't know how I would have felt if the CEO of Saint Thomas and my doctors would have told Barbara Kopple that what was important was the hospital's image, not filming the life and death struggle of a high-risk surgery. I will never know, but I am thankful for the hope that came from the team and the many who reached out with love.

— 14 —

Nigeria, West Africa, 1988

After my *Bloody Mary Morning* my life was completely changed. My priorities were different. My amazement at the goodness of my newfound faith and my confidence in the Lord was childlike. I could not get over the change in my heart, the excitement to awaken each morning with a prayer of Thanksgiving on my lips. With coffee in hand, I would go and sit in the bay window of my guest bedroom, and read the Bible. The Bible had always been a book of confusion for me, seemingly contradicting itself. Now, the words just seem to pop off the page at me and the meanings were deep and transforming. In the months that followed that January 1988 morning, I read the entire Bible, front to back and enjoyed it. Actually enjoyed it! The truths changed my thinking, my life.

I had no idea when I purchased that home that it would become a sanctuary of sorts for me. I purchased it from my friends, the builders, Dennis Brandon and Wayne Hilton. They had not mentioned the group that met regularly in the Club House. Though not all of the group lived in our complex, they were all members of Belmont Church on Nashville's Music Row, just a block from my office at ASCAP.

Neighbors who were members of that group had asked me many times to join them on Sunday evenings and I would always graciously respond with a "Thanks, if I can." But I never did. In fact, if I were home when they began to gather, I would turn out my lights and close my curtains, so they'd think I wasn't there. Of course, my car was just outside, and they knew I was there, but they never pushed. I guess they figured I would come when or if I was ready.

The morning after my Bloody Mary Morning was Sunday and I awoke that morning feeling like a million bucks. I showered and dressed and headed out the door for Belmont Church, which I had visited years before while in college at Lipscomb. Belmont was previously a Church of Christ that had recognized the Holy Spirit and began preaching about the Spirit. Working on Music Row, I had followed the growth of the church through the years but had not set foot within the doors for over 15 years. Belmont had grown too large for the small historic chapel on the corner of Music Row West and Grand Avenue, so they were meeting at West End Junior High School on West End Avenue just a few miles outside of downtown.

I parked my car and headed inside, greeting people along the way. I was excited to be in a church service again and looking forward to worshipping the God that I now knew existed. I walked into the auditorium and it was not difficult to find my neighbors and others in the group that met on Sunday evenings. I had heard that this group was praying for me, and yet, when they looked up and saw me standing at the head of the row that morning, they all looked amazingly surprised. I remember thinking and possibly asking them, *Where was the faith?* Had they not prayed that the Lord would touch my heart and bring me to Him? They not only made room for me on the row that morning but made room in their hearts for me in the weeks, months and years to come. I was, I am, so blessed to have been grafted into that family of believers in that first season of my Christian walk.

In addition to the Belmont home group, there were other believers like Barbi and Harlan Moore, who lived two doors from me. Harlan was on staff as the Worship Pastor of Nashville's First Church of the Nazarene on Woodland Street, just on the edge of downtown. His wife Barbi worked for I CARE Ministries, which is an acronym for International Christian Artists Reaching the Earth, a Ministry of singer-songwriter, Scott Wesley Brown. One morning as I went out to go to work, I saw Barbi in the parking lot in front of her condo, and she told me she had a unique opportunity she wanted to share with me. And little did I know, this *proposition* would further change my life.

Barbi was organizing a team to go to Benin City, Nigeria, West Africa for a week-long International Praise Conference and Worship Seminar. This event would be hosted by Church of God Mission in Benin City and attended by numerous worship teams and bands from not only Nigeria, but Ghana and other African nations. Teams of us Nashville musicians would teach seminars on various music topics. We also were excited to have Christian artists, like Danniebelle Hall, Babbie Mason, and Alvin Slaughter, perform during our evening concerts. Barbi asked if I would pray about going on that trip to help lead a group of background vocalists that would accompany the performing artists. Praying about a decision, now that was a new concept for me. Praying, asking GOD for wisdom and for His plan. Another life-changing concept in my newfound life of faith.

After talking with my new home group friends, and praying about it, I accepted her invitation. The trip was being planned for that coming summer. She then told me I might want to raise financial support for the trip, involving others, as partners, senders. Raise financial support, partners? That was also a new concept for me. I had never heard of that before, but I was open to whatever. So I created a newsletter blurb and sent it out to some friends and a few family members. I was pleasantly surprised and touched when my father said he wanted to make a donation to my trip.

Perhaps he saw me as worth investing in? That would be a new beginning in our relationship.

That summer in Nigeria, not only were there concerts by Scott Wesley Brown and other U.S. talents, but extremely popular Nigerian artists. There were also local bands and bands from the region of West Africa, as well as a very large choir that was directed by my neighbor, Harlan Moore. Wow! What a sound that choir produced! The round church building, the 3-tiered auditorium reverberated with voices praising the Creator. I will never forget when the choir led us in the old hymn, "Holy, Holy, Holy, Lord God Almighty." Every hair stood up on my arms and neck, and I was unable to utter a note. I was moved to tears as that hymn I had grown up singing in church rang out with so much enthusiasm. I think this was the first time those timeless lyrics actually popped out and meant something to me, to my faith. At that moment my heart was broken for the Lord, and maybe my soul was purchased for missions. I would never be the same again.

Another extremely moving time was when Babbie Mason performed her song "All Rise" which was one of the most-recorded contemporary Christian songs of the 1990s. Babbie's beautiful voice ringing out with the international choir, singing, praising! Wow, it was a picture of what heaven must be like.

"All rise, All rise, To stand before the throne in the presence of the Holy One"

"All rise, All rise, As we worship the Messiah, All rise!"

My mission trip to Nigeria was absolutely a fabulous experience. We had a great team of people traveling, and I enjoyed meeting and getting to know some amazing Africans during our week together. It was more than wonderful, I was so blessed to be part of that event.

On the return trip home, the I CARE staff offered a two-day stopover tourist package, allowing us to see a bit of London and

Amsterdam. Seven of us opted for those days and enjoyed the time to reflect and sightsee a bit in much cooler temperatures than in West Africa. Somewhere in my stack of photo albums is a picture of our team on one of those famous Amsterdam 1-hour canal cruises... fast asleep.

This was my first time in Europe. I had no idea that summer of '88, that in just a couple of years I would make Europe my home for nearly 25 years.

As wonderful as the trip was, it was nice to get home. I was tired but excited to tell all that I had experienced to anyone that would listen. But, soon enough, life went back to normal. I was enjoying my work on Music Row, my home, church group... I was living the dream. Was I? Well, not completely. I was still putting off signing the divorce papers. I knew the inevitable was coming and in early autumn I signed the papers and the divorce was final by November. In the end, we agreed to disagree. It was the right thing to do, but it was hard. I know that God dislikes divorce, however, there are circumstances in which we find ourselves, and God sees us through the darkness and forgives our failures. He helps us move forward, for which I am forever grateful.

1988 was a huge year of change... yes, there was some sadness and loss, but extreme joy. My Home Group had become like family and they loved me and discipled me well. With the new year of 1989 ringing in, I was blessed and content, yet my heart wanted more, as it seemed to be longing for purpose.

More was coming, and soon!

15

On The Cover of *Ad Age* Magazine

I do not remember having any doubts that the hospital would approve the filming of my surgery. When the Nashville hospital gave the green light to follow and film my case, it was like everybody on the hospital team and on the film crew had been infused with enthusiasm. In retrospect I believe creating a narrative of hope is fundamental to healthcare. Just think if every surgery were filmed for a docu-drama or a social media post. It might change the way everyone involved behaved. Research has proven that patients who are hopeful return to health more rapidly and have a higher rate of survival. Dr. Jerome Groopman, in his book *The Anatomy of Hope,* writes, "Instilling hope in the brain involves setting a firm goal and anticipating the reward of living with the dream fulfilled." I can't describe the role of the commercials in my surgery any better. Dr. Groopman's research proved that during a health crisis, *belief and expectation*—the two elements of hope—have an impact on the nervous system and this sets off a chain reaction that improves recovery. Sure, the dark hours of Cardiac Intensive Care were difficult. There was the breathing tube, the claustrophobia, but also the beauty of those who touched my life in those hard hours. I was a celebrity because the hospital had so much invested in me and my recovery, so I got excellent attention from all the staff. They made me feel like part of the team, not part of their workload for the day, which elevated my interaction with them. We were all part of a narrative of healing. Sure, Saint Thomas took a risk on my survival, but the risk paid off. I am surprised that there have not been more commercials like mine. What better way to champion a hospital than "… by showing competent professionals soberly going about their business," as *Ad Age* put it. That article in *Ad Age* goes on to say:

> *What distinguishes this campaign—and redeems it—is its understatement and restraint. To the credit of the advertiser and its agency, the selective truth is an unadorned truth. There is no suggestion, for instance, that Saint Thomas somehow takes the fear out of health crises or gives you better odds against death. Indeed, it rather chillingly documents how lucky this guy was to make it to surgery, much less through it.*

This was the genius of Barbara Kopple, no doubt. She knew how to tell a story, for it takes a good storyteller to create experiences that an audience can believe in and identify with. The commercials grew along with my healing, revealing moments of transformation that delighted employees as much as the they delighted me. One of these moments happened when Dr. Petracek told his staff to give me a little more time before giving me a blood transfusion, though two transfusions had been predicted prior to surgery. "Let's give him a little more time to see if his blood pressure will come back up on its own." It was another dramatic moment when my body did indeed respond on its own, and there would be no need for even one *transfusion*.

You only get this reality in commercials when hospitals raise the stakes and defy the norm. It only happens when you break the script.

Being filmed for commercials during one's most vulnerable hours would horrify some people, but it proved to be a welcome distraction for me and even my family and friends. The crew and the staff joined "my team" as they created hope and the feeling of being on a larger team pulling for one ultimate goal—my survival.

But I've always believed that God had more for me to do in my life than to end it in that lake in Holland, in Budapest, the flights home, or in surgery at Saint Thomas Hospital. I believe Michael Petracek was right when he said, "The Lord must surely have his hand on this young man. This tear is huge... I can't believe he survived it."

So did I need those commercials? I do not really know, but I believe that God ordained them. Everything lined up perfectly for them to be filmed.

Maybe this is a theme that I have experienced throughout my life. I now believe that even through the hard times, God was there with me. He takes all of our experiences, talents, successes and failures and uses them to mold us closer to His likeness. I think this step-by-step guidance led me into world missions and later becoming a pastor.

16

All The Vain Things That
Charm Me Most

I love Christmas and the festive nature of the season, the songs, the lights, the trees, the food, the parties. It is truly like the song says, "It's the Most Wonderful Time of the Year." I usually get my Christmas tree and decorate it on the Friday after the American holiday, Thanksgiving, and it stays up until New Year's Day and sometimes a bit after. But the Christmas of 1988 was even more special as it was my first Christmas to celebrate the birth of Christ with the actual belief that there was a birth and He did come to the earth, and for me, for my salvation!

Music Row pretty much shuts down the last two weeks of the year. If our offices were open then we were just enjoying office parties and hanging out with friends, coworkers and colleagues from The Row. Just before the holidays I received a call from Barbi Moore asking if I would come over to her office for a meeting with her and Steve Lorenz. By December of '88 I was very familiar with the Lorenz building that housed the office for I CARE. Since our summer mission trip, Steve and Marilyn Lorenz had become part of my extended family.

Once there, Barbi and Steve started talking about our recent trip to Benin City and all the amazing feedback they had received from that trip. We swapped a number of warm memories and it was fun reminiscing with them. Pretty quickly they came to the point of our meeting by asking me this question: "Would you consider becoming I CARE's West Africa Director?" That would require moving to Nigeria summer of '89 to prepare for the praise and worship conference, January '90.

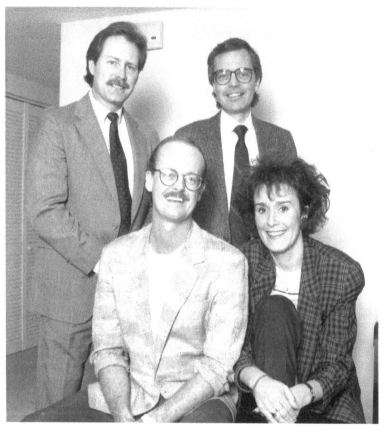

Sheila Walsh, Tom Long and Steve Lorenz
Photo: 1989 Alan L Mayor

They went on to explain there was no salary offered by I CARE, this would be a full-time mission career where I would raise my own support. What? Wait! Did I understand that you want me to quit my cushy gig at ASCAP, leave my home, my friends and family, my life, AND raise my own salary? From where? From whom? From what? Raising support for a mission trip was one thing, but raising support to live? Hmm, I thought... "Someone is crazy here... either them or me". So after they made their pitch, and I took a few minutes appropriate for ponder, I politely declined, thanked them and left, and that was it. Over, or so I thought.

The holidays were full of the excitement of Christmas and yet there was something missing in my soul. My heart was amiss. I remember being my *party self* on the outside, but something was not quite right on the inside. I was longing for the purpose I had felt when we were in Nigeria with all of those amazing African people. The happiest, most joyful people that I had ever seen, even though most had so little in material wealth.

Though I loved my West African experience, some of the sights and smells in the areas of toilets and sewage were almost more than I could handle. Public toilets were almost nonexistent at that time and therefore people were forced to do their business wherever they could. I understood after entering a few public restrooms why the men just went on the back walls of the nearest buildings.

Sometimes, walking through the open markets, I would encounter odors that were not pleasing to my sensitive sense of smell. At times one might need to be careful where one stepped walked due to the lack of facilities. Again, the challenges of Africa, and yet, the happiest people I had ever been around. And during the holiday season of '88 those smells started to come back to me. But as opposed to a negative feeling, there was something positive in the memories. I was experiencing a sense of longing, a desire to be back there, back with the people. My heart was being drawn back to Africa. I cannot explain that other than to say it was yet another God moment in my life.

I could not get these memories, sights, and smells out of my mind. I continued to work, see my friends, go to church, but something was missing. Something was lacking—or was it fear? I had been raised in religion, I have often said that we were the *Frozen Chosen* in the church. I had grown up seeing bench warmers and I wanted more than that. I had experienced this amazing change, this amazing touch by God, and I did not want that to end. I wanted all of God that I could have. I wanted more than a Sunday morning seat in a church; I wanted to share the Love and Hope that I had experienced just a year before on that Bloody Mary Morning.

One Wednesday afternoon in late winter of '89, after work, I decided to go down the street to Belmont Church for their Wednesday evening service. By this time, Belmont was meeting in the new building on Music Row.

On that particular Wednesday evening they were singing when I arrived, and Dr. Don Finto, the senior pastor, was overseeing the service. After I took my seat, the worship leader began to sing the beautiful old hymn, "When I Survey the Wondrous Cross," which was a favorite of mine.

Just as we were about to sing verse two, Pastor Don jumped up from the front row and in typical Don fashion asked everyone to stop singing. He wanted us to weigh out the words that we were about to sing, and he urged us not to sing the verse unless we really meant those words, really meant to sacrifice! The lyrics of the second verse read, *Forbid it, Lord, that I should boast, save in the death of Christ my Lord. All the vain things that charm me most, I sacrifice them to His blood.* As I sat there contemplating these words, I realized that it was the vain things that charmed me, the vain things that were keeping me from answering this call to missions and accepting the I CARE position and moving to West Africa. That was why my heart was so unsettled over the past few months. I longed for that purpose I had found on my mission trip that past summer. I was *supposed* to be a missionary! I sang that second verse through tears. I knew that I would be leaving my home, my job, my friends and family. I was embarking on a new career of which I had never dreamed!

I had no concept of raising money to support myself. Who would I ask for money and why would they give me their hard-earned money? It was a totally new idea, a new concept, and I needed time to understand it. I thought maybe I should talk to people who lived that way. At the time I didn't know anyone who lived on support, so I thought maybe my church would give, especially since I was going abroad to do the Lord's work. I mean, Scripture says the church will. Right? Or does it?

I remember a good friend telling me, once I had decided to move to Nigeria, that I should not expect to ever own a house again, meaning I could not own a house because missionaries just don't do that. Meaning that missionaries are poor. A few years later at a Missions Conference a woman told me how much she admired missionaries. She went on to explain it was because of the commitment, but also for "taking a vow of poverty." Poverty? Did I take such a vow?

Even as I agreed in my new found faith and excitement, to accept this career change and began to learn about raising financial support, somewhere in the back of my mind I wondered why missionaries 'should' be poor, not have a home. I was used to seeing pastors living normal lives, in nice homes, some well above *normal* in almost palatial homes. I wondered why it should be so different. Surely if we are *all called* to live for Christ and do His will, then leaving home and family to serve Him in a foreign land, especially a third world country, surely the Church, His Church, His people would rally behind missionaries and give of their means in order to send them. I thought we were all in this together. When I read the Bible, it said GO into all the world and preach the Gospel (Matthew 28:19-20). I thought that was a mandate for us all.

Was I really going to quit my job at ASCAP? Was I prepared to move across the world and live in a third world country? Prepared? Most definitely not!

Despite being so unprepared, God used that move in such an incredible way in my life. I have found that is the nature of God, His mysterious ways. He uses our obedience, even without proper training, so that He is glorified in the end. God does so much in us, and yes, even through us.

17

Checkpoint Charlie, East Berlin, 1989

The spring before my move to Nigeria, I was introduced to Eastern Europe. On a return planning trip to Nigeria, Barbi, Steve and I had a two-day layover in West Berlin. We were there to meet with German born Evangelist, Reinhard Bonnke, and Peter Vandenberg (Vice President, Christ For All Nations). During our meeting, we discussed ministry in West Africa, with a special focus on our mutual work in Nigeria. Bonnke attracted massive crowds in Africa during decades of preaching and is said to have changed the face of Christianity in Africa.

The second day, Sunday, we set out from our hotel in brightly colored West Berlin for the infamous "Checkpoint Charlie," crossing into Communist East Berlin. The guards were very serious, ordering us to empty our pockets and backpacks for a thorough search. We complied in every way, of course, as our goal was to be admitted, to meet a couple in the East side of the city. On the opposite side of the guard gate, surrounded by high barbed wire walls; there was no color. It was as if we had crossed into the Land of Oz in reverse—from full technicolor to black and white. The streets were dirty, not from trash, but from coal soot and lack of care. There was little grass in the green spaces, and what grassy areas that did exist were unkept and mostly weeds.

Through a mutual friend we had a prearranged meeting point with the couple, and they led us to their flat. Inside the apartment, we were quickly warmed by their hospitality and kindness. We had some food and fellowship before going to the recording studio hidden in the church basement. If caught, they could face prison time for producing what was considered contraband and Christian propaganda. This couple informed us that due to their Christianity, they were paid less than their contemporaries. Spending time with these lovely people who cared so much for their fellowmen, their Christian brothers and sisters, and their love for the Lord, made a lasting impression on my heart.

As the day was coming to a close, we said our goodbyes and began our walk back to Checkpoint Charlie. Our host walked with us, but stopped a few blocks away from the border. He said going further could put him under suspicion for even being seen with westerners. So we said one more goodbye, and quietly made our way back across the small but huge divide between East and West Berlin.

On the flight back to the States, the next day, I was processing the devastation of the Cold War, The East Bloc, and what a city divided by a wall meant for both sides. It forever changed my life. But later that year, that wall, the Berlin Wall was torn down by politically imprisoned people.

I was living in Nigeria when I got my first information about the destruction of the wall. I had traveled into Lagos for an overnight trip to speak and sing at a church when I stopped for a nice *western meal* at the Lagos Sheraton Hotel. While in their bookshop, I picked up a magazine with a picture of the Brandenburg Gate. It was covered with people sitting and climbing on the wall... with tools to hammer away at a 50-year prison. I was dumbstruck.

The Wall was a monument to evil. I remember turning to a well-dressed westerner, probably an international businessman, and asked if this was true or some kind of a spoof magazine, fake news. He looked at me with suspicion and responded with a German accent, "Yes, of course it is real, where have you been?"

I had been raised by an authoritarian father, where it was simply not okay to be different. I had to conform to what was thought to be "normal" by others, and my dreams were squelched. These things had been part of my childhood and were certainly *the norm* in communist Europe. So my heart opened to them, as they opened themselves to the world. I wanted to support the people and the local church, which had survived—miraculously in some cases. Due to persecution many pastors had been imprisoned at some point, for their faith.

I knew when I came out of East Berlin that night through Checkpoint Charlie that I was somehow, somewhere, sometime going to work with these neglected people... I could relate to them.

— 18 —

Oyinbo

My Home Group had been a refuge and place to grow during that first year and a half, since I had asked Jesus into my heart. As I was newly divorced, my friends at the condominium complex in Nashville became my Christian family. We enjoyed being together, discussing the sermon that we had heard on Sunday at church simply enjoying a meal together. Lots of laughter and lots of care. We prayed for each other and for the challenges in life we faced. We were committed to walk together through these challenges of life. We had older more settled people and younger couples with young children, and we were close.

Their influence was much like a story I heard about an African who was told by an early missionary that water sometimes became so hard that someone could walk on it. He said he believed a great many things the missionary had told him, but he never would believe that. When he came to England as a guest of the missionary, it came to pass that one cold day he saw the river frozen, but he would not venture on it. He knew that it was a deep river, and he felt certain that he would be drowned. No matter how much coaxing he would not walk on the frozen water until the missionary and his friends did. Then he was persuaded and trusted himself where others had safely ventured. This is what the home group did for me. They taught me how to venture out away from my shame and guilt, and trust myself with Christ. If not for their support, I might not have gone to Nigeria on that first trip, summer of '88.

They sent me off and shared in the joy upon my return, patiently looking at the photos and listening to the stories. I know they were not prepared for my announcement and my move to Nigeria less than a year later, but then, neither was I.

I began the process of packing up and asking friends to take items to their homes for storage for a time. Good friends took my very large, antique dining room furniture which ended up being used in five homes over the following 15 years. Another friend took my grand piano that I had owned since my home in Historic Edgefield. There were lots of little things I gave away and some things just ended up at the local thrift store. It was hard and yet freeing to some degree to begin this new life of missions and ministry. Truly, my vain things were being removed or loaned out.

As I packed up two trunks and a couple of suitcases, I remember lining the trunks with rolls of toilet paper. I removed the flimsy cardboard tube and mashed the toilet paper roll as thin as possible. This padded the sides so that the desktop computer, monitor, and keyboard could travel safely. It worked, and I had *western* toilet paper for the entire time I was in Nigeria! And probably gifted plenty of rolls to other missionaries when I left. You can't know what these little gifts mean to ex pats. They are a touch of home.

The day came for my move. As I left the condo that morning, I remember being excited and scared to death at the same time. I knew that friends and family would come to the Nashville airport that morning to see me off. That was going to be fun and hard. Back then, prior to 9/11 in America, you could go to the gate to see your friends off. I forget how many people came to the airport that morning, but it was a sizable number. I have photos of dozens of people gathered at the gate to talk, laugh, cry, and to pray for me. It was an emotional moment when I waved my final wave to my father who was there with his portable oxygen tank. Even though my father and I had challenges in our relationship, he did love me. He was proud of me, I think, but that was mixed with fear for me to be so far away. Dad would rarely ever say that he was proud of me or my brothers, though I remember seeing pride in his eyes at times. He struggled with his own self-worth and identity, which made it hard for him to affirm others, especially his own sons. Despite the challenges, I was glad he was there. We shared a hug that morning, and I told him that I loved him. I wish now I had taken a few more minutes with him. All too quickly we were boarding, and then I was seated on the plane. I turned to the window and cried.

Flying out of Nashville that morning was hard for me even though I had a strong sense of purpose and excitement as I embarked on this new season of my life. It was prearranged that I would meet Dr. Mark and Doreen Babo, in the Boston, Massachusetts airport for a short layover before the overnight flight to Amsterdam. Mark and Doreen were starting a clinic in Benin City. The next two flights were long but I was young enough to find it exciting. Approximately eight hours to Amsterdam, a five hour layover, and then another seven hours to Nigeria. We landed in Lagos around midnight... exhausted!

One of the things I remember about arriving in Nigeria is off-boarding the plane. Even before the seatbelt signs were turned off, everyone would jump up, grab their luggage from the overhead bins, cram themselves into the aisle, to wait. While you were waiting, laden with bags and crammed together without an inch to spare, you heard the jet engines shut down. Within seconds, you felt the humidity. The heat from the equator-climate engulfed the plane. Immediately you started to perspire, droplets of sweat began to run down your body under your shirt and trousers. Once through Passport Control, you enter the large Lagos Airport Terminal. Your senses immediately assaulted by the throng of people. Passengers looking for family, taxi drivers wanting to find fares, touts who want to carry your luggage, for a fee. Some of these touts were aggressive, grabbing at your luggage before you have had a chance to acclimate to the chaos. Thankfully, when Mark, Doreen and I arrived there was someone from Church of God Mission there to collect us. Somehow they found us, gathered up our bags and as quickly as possible moved us through this ocean of people. Once inside the small transport bus, we felt a sense of relief. This was my third arrival in Murtala Muhammed International Airport in a year, so I was starting to get a bit accustomed to the process. Nevertheless, I was glad to be inside the minibus.

In my previous two arrivals we had driven to a local hotel, had a snack, then at least a few hours of sleep. The following morning, we would enjoy a nice breakfast in the hotel before the journey to Benin City, almost 6 hours by road. But on this arrival, one of our hosts wanted to get back quickly so it was decided that we would drive through the night. This would be our second night in a row without sleep. Since we were hungry, our hosts stopped at a roadside food vendor that had some small items over an open flame, a piece of corn and a drink. It was our only option, so we purchased our little *To Go* meals and quickly were back on the bus before a harrowing road trip to Benin City. There were military checkpoints along the way and each time they had to shine their torches (flashlights) on our passports and then on our faces. There was always a play for a bribe, but our hosts were seasoned and strong and if there were bribes paid, I was unaware of them. It was morning before we arrived at the Church of God Mission compound on Airport Road in Benin City. I was assigned to be the guest of a British family who came down from their apartment to collect me and take me into their home. I was able to get a few more hours of sleep before awaking with food poisoning, at worst, or some ugly bacteria, at best. Needless to say, I felt like a human fountain... not pretty. My hosts, whom I had met the summer before but did not know, kindly brought me a cool glass bottle of sugar water to sip to keep me hydrated until the *water works* stopped. I was so sick, and so far from home. What had I done?

A few days later, restored to health, I moved out of the compound and just down the street to join Mark and Doreen in the house appointed for them to live. It was a simple stucco style bungalow with hot pink interior walls. Seems like the tile floor had more golds in it, no sign of pink in the floor that I can remember. There was only one thing in the house and that was a small gas stove with four cooking burners on top. The cooking hobs were covered with a glass protective top, or so we thought. Once lit, that glass rose to a temperature that eventually exploded with glass going everywhere in that kitchen. Thankfully, Doreen, Mark and I were in the living room when the explosion shook the house. Oh well, so much for the one nice item in the house. Guess that glass top was meant to be removed before one lit the gas eyes.

Despite the dark hot pink walls and the lack of furniture, Mark, Doreen and I made our first days in the house quite fun. One day we heard of a woman nearby who made loaves of bread and sold them first come first serve in the community. We jumped into 'our' old Peugeot loaner and set out to find her, to purchase a few loaves of fresh soft bread, some butter, then feasted until we were so very full. We also located furniture, I believe, within the compound and began to furnish Mark and Doreen's house.

After a couple of weeks, word came from the ministry office that my apartment was ready for me to move into. I had already ordered a bed be made from a local carpenter and had purchased a mattress in a local shop. The bed was all that I had. The building was a block away, outside of the compound walls. When I arrived, I realized that I was the only resident. There were three additional apartments, but empty. My first night sleeping in my new bed in a four-unit house where I was the only human was maybe a bit daunting. I was not convinced that I was safe in that house alone on that dirt road leading into the fields. I also missed Mark and Doreen.

Within a few days of attempting to settle into my new digs, I heard a rumor that one of the westerners was leaving, and therefore, his apartment might be free. That apartment was inside the compound, on the 3rd floor with a small balcony. It was also furnished, and I immediately went to my host, Archbishop Benson Idahosa, and politely requested that flat/apartment. He granted my wish, and very quickly, I was settled into my new home.

Within a few weeks of arrival I experienced something that I had not experienced since my childhood, and then only once. Homesickness! I am not talking about a bit of loneliness and maybe some sadness. I am talking about full on homesick, extreme sadness, bordering on depression. I was sad and full of regret, I wanted home. Like a child; I just wanted to go home. I didn't struggle so much in the daylight hours when I was around others, but in the evenings when I closed the door to my flat, tossing and turning through the long warm nights. However, I always felt a bit brighter in the mornings. During that period, I would sit, thinking of home, in front of my electric fan, well… on the evenings that electricity worked. The National Electric Power Authority (NEPA) was most undependable. When it went off, and that fan stopped, I would sink into despair, another night on top of the sheets just praying for even the slightest breeze. My homesickness got so bad that I started telling myself before bed, that if I do not feel better in the morning, I am packing up, going down the street to the Benin City airport, boarding a plane to Lagos… and then home! However, mornings came, it was cooler, and each morning there was a bit more hope in my heart.

I honestly do not remember how many of those early weeks I felt so homesick, but it was at least a few. Then, as quickly as it came, it left. I remember one evening thinking, *Wait, I haven't felt homesick in days.* I was over it. I am thankful to say that I never experienced homesickness again. I have since lived in many places, apartments and houses in foreign lands and I have adjusted quickly and without any sadness or hopeless adjustments.

As a new Christian, and a very independent American, I sometimes pushed the boundaries of safety. There were road bandits on the highways in Nigeria, and yet on occasion I would get into my old Peugeot and drive myself, alone in my car the six hours to Lagos, or two and a half hours to Warri or even a 12-hour drive north to Jos. What was I thinking?

On one of those trips to Lagos I found myself on the motorway snaking through that massive city. My destination was the Sheraton Hotel, but driving after dark I was unable to make out the road signs. I am not sure where I was in the city, I just remember being on a flyover on the inside lane of 3 lanes. In my rearview mirror, I saw a group of young men running alongside of cars trying to get money from drivers. The traffic was bumper-to-bumper and moving very slowly. The group was getting closer—I was trapped. One of the men yelled, "Oyinbo." (Oyinbo was their word for Caucasian, European, non-African, which communicates, *rich*.) At that moment the entire group followed the man who yelled, and ran for my car. Just as I thought, *God help me*, the cars in the two lanes to my right literally stopped. That created a 40-degree angle of open road. I turned my wheel and sped across those two lanes. To my amazement, there was a ramp exiting the flyover, leading down into the dark city. I was lost and alone, but at least it was dark. No one could see that I was an Oyinbo.

The darkness made navigating very difficult so I found what looked to be a decent hotel and went in. They were as surprised to see me approach the counter as I was to be there. I said that I needed a room for the night, and they gave me a room key and I headed upstairs to find the dimly lit room. Once inside, I locked the door and took a straight chair and wedged it under the doorknob. That was a long and sleepless night. Someone, or multiple people, tried to get into my room the entire night. Just when I dozed off, in hopes of sleep, the door would begin to rattle again, sometimes with great force. I am thankful for that old wooden chair that kept these potential intruders at bay. The morning came, I checked out and found the Sheraton, took a shower and enjoyed a good meal. Through the years, I have reflected upon this story many times. This was another God moment!

As traumatic as that night was, it still did not prevent me from driving alone in Nigeria. Sometimes I just needed to get away. In developing countries when you are white or western of any shade, you are considered rich. You are! I was! Even on minimal financial support, I was still rich in comparison. Having an American or any first world passport automatically makes one rich. Rich, because we have opportunities that one simply does not have in the impoverished or developing nations.

As a westerner, a rich person in Nigeria, it was expected you have house help. I was a single man living in a two-bedroom, one-bathroom apartment with a kitchen and a living-dining room combo, and yet I was expected to have a cleaning girl, a woman or girl to wash my clothes and do my ironing. You must iron everything due to worm larvae that can penetrate your skin simply from hanging on the clothesline to dry. I also had a driver at my disposal and a cook. All of my house help attended the Bible school next door to our compound. They were all lovely young people, and I was happy to help them by employing them even a few hours each day or week. I was not happy, however, that my little apartment was like Grand Central Station. Sometimes I just wanted to read a book or play some music without all the comings and goings, but I still enjoyed it for the most part. I did really enjoy the young man who came a few times a week to cook for me. He was from Ghana, a neighboring West African country, and he made the best pepe chicken and rice. It was spicy and I love spicy food. I would sit and eat, then wipe my brow, then eat some more. Between the spicy pepe chicken and the hot humidity of the region, I was always warm.

A couple of times, to get a break from the heat, I drove almost 12 hours north to the higher elevation of Jos. Jos was the home of an international high school where missionaries and business-people sent their children to school. It was a lovely campus and they had lots of activities including an evening where we learned Scottish dances. I enjoyed speaking at the school assemblies and hanging out with the teachers and students. The cool air added to my enjoyment of those visits, but I still marvel at the insanity to have driven so far alone.

Closer to Benin City is the smaller city of Warri. Early on I had met Rick and Donna Whitcomb, who at that time lived in Warri, Delta State. I had the pleasure of visiting them and their children a number of times. Most visits, I drove there alone as well. In autumn of 1989 German evangelist Reinhard Bonnke did an evangelistic crusade in Warri. As you may remember from an earlier chapter, I had been to Berlin for meetings with the Bonnke people prior to moving to Nigeria, so it was a pleasure for me to connect with the Bonnke Crusade pre-team. I was impressed with their pre-preparations for this huge event. I was also glad to see Peter Vandenberg again whom I had met in Berlin. Peter was the driver of my first high-speed-spin on the German Autobahn.

I was also very impressed with Reinhard Bonnke himself in the few days we spent together in Warri. I had the pleasure of having lunch with him at the Whitcombs' home. During our discussions of life, he asked me to sing at the crusade one evening. That was another amazing experience and highlight in my life. Standing on that stage, faces as far as I could see literally blending into the night, and I was about to sing a solo for all of those amazing African people. What a great memory and what a blessing. Another God moment!

The autumn season of 1989 turned out to be one of the hardest-turned greatest times in my life. I learned so much about me, about the faithfulness of God and His people. I am honored to have lived in Nigeria, honored to have a place in my heart for Africa and its people. I was completely unprepared for my move into missions and ministry, yet God put some amazing people in my path to help me, to teach me, or to just support and love me as I began my mission career. It is impossible to thank everyone by name that I encountered in those days, but just know that I do carry each of you in my heart.

Christmas of 1989 was my first Christmas away from family and my homeland. I was expecting it to be a difficult day, but we had such a good time creating our celebrations that I got through it with minimal sadness or homesickness. Mark, Doreen and I created a symphony of pop bottles filled with different levels of water creating a music scale. A wonderful young lady named Laurie, who had joined Mark and Doreen at the clinic, played the fourth part. The four of us blew into those bottles playing Christmas songs and some hymns, however, I must admit the slightest awkward over-blow or weird sound could send us into laughter, making it almost impossible to get your lips back into the correct position, embouchure, as it were.

The first few days of January 1990, the I CARE team arrived from the States. We met in Lagos and transported them by bus to Benin City. Our conference would be hosted for the second year at Church of God Mission. The church was founded by Archbishop Benson Idahosa. He was a strong man whom God had used mightily in Nigeria. He was a powerful speaker, a strong leader, and was kind and hospitable to me in those months I lived in his compound.

During I CARE's Christian Artist Seminars, we worked with some wonderful musicians. Some from West African countries in the area, but most of them from Nigeria. A number of young bands and artists came for training purposes, as we offered workshops and seminars daily for artists, instrumentalists, and songwriters. Some were unknown to the public but were worship leaders in their churches. We also hosted concerts by well-known Nigerian artists like Chief Ebenezer Obey, a recording artist celebrity since the '50s and Panam Percy Paul from Jos in Plateau State.

At the end of our events, I traveled with the team back to Lagos to assist in seeing them safely to the airport for their return to the States. Then we, the leadership team, flew north to Jos for a few days of meetings and retreat. Afterwards we returned to Lagos for one final night together before they flew home to Nashville. The next morning I began the renewal process for my Nigerian visa. In just a few days my six-month visa would expire. Believe me you did not want to outstay your visa, your legal welcome.

A friend of our ministry and a pastor of one of the Lagos churches took my passport and went to the officials in Lagos requesting an additional six-month stamp. I waited. Thankful that I did not have to go in person, I waited in the Lagos Sheraton hotel that always hosted our arriving teams. It had a lovely restaurant with an international chef and the very best lasagna I have ever eaten. To this day it makes my mouth water just to think of it. The hotel had a pool, friendly staff, and great security, so I was good. The only negative was the hotel was not cheap, especially on a mission budget. I waited confidently that my visa extension would be renewed. On the last day of my visa, the pastor returned with my passport and said that they had denied our request. I had to leave the country. Now! Tonight! I needed to be on that last

KLM flight out of Lagos later that evening. Thankfully I still had a return ticket. I grabbed my bags and off to the Lagos airport we went. That airport at the time was known as one of the most corrupt airports in the world. Caution signs hung in other airports warning travelers to beware of flying through Lagos.

I went to the KLM counter and requested a seat on the fight that evening. There was a seat avilable, and I breathed a sigh of relief, since there was no Plan B. I got my boarding pass, said goodbye to the pastor who had brought me, and began moving toward Passport Control. I got to the checkpoint where they check your bags and documents before you would be allowed to enter the international section. I gave my passport to the guard and he said, "Your visa has expired, it expired today." I responded politely but confidently that it does not expire until midnight. He did not agree and called a couple of his colleagues over to discuss this situation with them. Each of them tried to tell me the same, that my visa was expired and that I needed to go back to the government tomorrow and get it approved to either stay or permission to leave.

I wasn't super well-educated in corruption at that point, though I had learned quite a lot after living there and witnessing the bribe culture in the planning and execution of the I CARE event, so I was wise enough. I dislike injustice, and can be stubborn when I feel like I am being cheated. I refused the temptation to *grease their palms*, to pay the bribe they were obviously wanting. Nothing was said about a bribe, of course, but I knew. I decided to bluff and continued to move with the line toward the metal detectors and final checkpoint. I just kept telling the officers who stayed beside me that my visa was good until midnight. My brain was not nearly as confident as my posture, I was praying constantly that God would once again open a door for me. When we reached the machine, I gathered all of my confidence in the Lord, and said to them directly my visa is good, please move aside and let me pass and I will be out of the country before midnight. They then motioned me over to a curtained off area where they would frisk those suspected of concealing something. The three men surrounded me in that small space and began to physically hand frisk me. I have been frisked before in a number of airports and checkpoints including the Amsterdam airport, but this was intended to intimidate me. They put their hands under my shirt, pressing into me, trying to make me afraid... I just refused to react. I just prayed silently that the Lord would protect me and keep me strong and I kept my eyes locked on theirs; they grew weary and moved away, allowing me to pass into the international wing. Another God moment.

I was so happy to be in that humid, badly lit corridor, where at least I knew I was getting on that KLM flight and would be in the sky, headed to London before my visa expired at midnight.

19

Musicians For Missions, Amsterdam

I CARE Founder, Scott Wesley Brown, had suggested that I stop over in England on my way home from Africa. He wanted me to meet his friend Lynn Green. Lynn was the leader of the YWAM work located in Harpenden, just a few miles north of London.

Harpenden's Hospitality rooms were in a cozy old English tutor style house on the Highfield Oval. England was cool and rainy, and I was tired of heat and sunshine so I slept very well that evening. The next day I met with Lynn and after some discussion, mostly about music and missions, he suggested that I fly to the Netherlands to meet Karen Lafferty. Karen is the Founder and Director of YWAM's Musicians for Missions (MFM), based in Amsterdam at that time.

It might be good to note that, *once upon a time*, and *not so long ago*, you could change your flights without a problem or added charges, as long as you were going the same direction. The next morning I trained back to London and flew across the Channel to Amsterdam.

Upon arrival at Schiphol International Airport I was met by a YWAM'er and driven to one of the their ministry buildings, De Poort, in the heart of Amsterdam. I was welcomed and shown to a lovely room in De Poort's hospitality wing. De Poort was a repurposed seamen's dormitory house that was built in the 1800s. YWAM has a high value for hospitality and most bases have some rooms always available for speakers, supporters, and traveling guests. I was enjoying my lovely hospitality room overlooking the canal and the Scheepvaart Museum. I slept so well.

The dining hall in De Poort seemed to always be full of students and staff. International students of all ages gathered for their six-month Discipleship Training School. DTS byline: "To Know God and Make Him Known."

Our meals were always in community and everyone pitched in to either cook or clean up afterwards; either way there was lots of good conversations and fellowship.

The first full day there I met with Karen Lafferty. She told me that on Friday evening there was going to be a concert of talents within the schools and asked if I would like to stay over for that. I did and it was fun and meaningful evening. I even performed a Larry Gatlin song, representing Nashville and country.

She also asked if I would like to travel with her and a friend to another YWAM Base in Holland, in Heidebeek an hour and a half east. There we would celebrate the birthday of one of the MFM staff, Cathy Carter. So I said "Sure", I was always up for an adventure and meeting people.

The next morning, after breakfast, we loaded up in Karen's Peugeot estate car (station wagon) and headed out on our day trip. When we arrived, the DTS class had just taken a break for lunch and about to sing "Happy Birthday" to Cathy. I was only in Amsterdam a few days on that trip, but made what would become a number of life long friends.

There were Summer of Service (SOS) outreaches being planned with Go-Teams, for the following summer. A number of ministry trips and teams traveling into the newly opened borders of the former Soviet Bloc. MFM Staff, Tim Berlin, Cathy Carter and Emmy Armbruster were creating a band called Frontrunner and asked if I would join them. The plan was to rehearse for a month, do some local outreach there, in Amsterdam, before joining with a larger team. In July we would travel across Germany, Austria and Hungary before reaching our destinations of Romania and Bulgaria, where we would spend 3 weeks ministering on the streets and in churches. We planned to return through what was then The Socialist Federal Republic of Yugoslavia. (SFRY) Specifically, the 6 republics that made up the federation were Bosnia and Herzegovina, Croatia, Macedonia, Montenegro, Serbia (including the regions of Kosovo and Vojvodina) and Slovenia. One year after our time there, on 25 June, 1991, the declarations of independence of Slovenia and Croatia effectively ended SFRY's existence.

I had dreamed of returning to the former East Bloc since my Berlin crossing through Checkpoint Charlie, spring of '89. I knew in my heart that day in Lagos, when I saw the photos of the Berlin Wall being dismantled, I would go there and minister.

I flew out of Amsterdam a day later to return to Nashville. Upon arrival, late that evening, I was met by an estimated 80 people, chanting my name. I was seated in the back of the plane, so I was last off, but I could hear them chanting when I began my walk down the jetway. Some of the passengers who had exited earlier had waited around to see who this famous person must be. One of those passengers actually broke through my hugging friends, to shake my hand.

It was a grand reunion as most of the crowd drove from the airport to Wayne and Pat Hilton's home that evening for a *Welcome Home Party*. This large group of friends made me feel so loved, they were happy to have me home. I was happy to be home, but I knew that I would be returning to Amsterdam and on to Eastern Europe very soon.

20

Smuggling Behind The Iron Curtain

I returned home to Nashville in February of 1990 and spent the next few months meeting and prayerfully considering my next step in missions. Even though I had enjoyed my West African experience, the challenges had been great, yet I had learned so much. But with the decline of an extended Nigerian visa, it seemed that this season had come to an end. I knew that post-communist Europe would be my niche.

As summer approached, I grew more and more excited about returning to Amsterdam and becoming part of the band, Frontrunner. There were a number of bands in MFM at that time, and they were using music to reach people in the city. There were different genres, and yet, we all enjoyed our fellowship and the community of people who made up YWAM-Amsterdam. Tim, Mary Vance, and their son, Boone, took me in to live in their third-floor bedroom in Zaandam, a bit north of Amsterdam. Sometimes we took Tim's car into the city for our rehearsals, but more often we rode the bus. This had its challenges, especially when carrying musical equipment like guitars and amps. One morning we were late leaving the house and just about to miss the bus when Tim yelled "RUN," so off we ran laden with equipment. I think the driver must have seen the crazy pair running, and decided to have mercy on us. He waited, which was most unusual. When we climbed aboard, huffing and puffing, every eye was on us and the amount of equipment we were hauling. The expressions on the reserved Dutch people's faces, made us laugh all the way into the city.

Frontrunner rehearsed every day in the Radar-Room, on the roof of the YWAM De Poort building. We began each morning with prayer for this beautiful city. In contrast to the gorgeous architecture and canals, it was also known for prostitution and drugs. Our goal, as a band, was to reach people with the hope conveyed in our music.

We were ultimately a vocal band with Tim and Mary Ellen playing guitars. Cathy and I were there to sing and harmonize and occasionally to play keyboard. In addition to our Christian songs we wanted a fun set of oldies… easy songs that people would remember from their past. Something that would make them smile. So we came up with a 50s medley.

We were surprised how much Europeans loved American 50s bebop songs. They even knew the words! The medley was always a hit wherever we sang.

Every Friday evening YWAM Amsterdam staff met as a community for a time of worship and community business. Frontrunner had been asked to lead worship, and we gladly accepted the opportunity. We opened the evening meeting with a number of well-known choruses and everyone joined in. After the speaker, and some announcements we were asked to come back to the stage for a closing song. Tim quietly whispered, "Should we do our 50s medley?" I was the new person, the *new kid on the block* and immediately was afraid that this would go over badly-given the serious and worshipful atmosphere. But who was I to say no? I saw Cathy and Emmy's eyes light up and the next second Tim put his baritone voice to the mic and started singing, *One, two, three o'clock, four o'clock, rock.* Just as we had rehearsed it, each of us added our harmony until we reached the *Let's Rock Around the Clock Tonight* —there was no turning back. Within seconds, the room erupted into song. The chairs quickly disappeared and the crowd was standing, singing, laughing, dancing—having a great time. What a fun memory!

The leader for our trip to Eastern Europe was Sverker Weissglas. (Say that 6 times or even once, if you are not Swedish.) Sverker was a charismatic leader with piercing dark eyes and a great smile. He could probably charm the skin off of a snake.

As our summer outreach began, our first day of travel took us from Amsterdam across Germany, Austria and to the Hungarian border. At that time there were still armed border crossings between Germany and Austria, and a very old soviet-style border crossing collection of buildings between Austria and Hungary. The Hungarian border was a fortress, complete with guard shacks on stilts, with men holding machine guns. Our entire bus was searched, and every passport presented and stamped, before we were allowed to cross into Hungary. A long night, but we finally stopped a couple of hours later in downtown Budapest on Margit Sziget (Margaret Island) in the middle of the Duna River (Danube). We slept the rest of the night in our seats awakening the next morning on this beautiful island. Our bus was parked in front of the Thermal Bath Hotel.

Mineral baths are thought to be one of the reasons the Romans settled in this area. Throughout the 16th and 17th centuries, Hungary was under the rule of the Ottoman Empire and Turkish style bathhouses were constructed in the city. Several remain standing today. One of those is the Király Fürdő. Known for its medieval Turkish architecture and octagonal dome roof, the Kiraly, (constructed in 1565 AD) was once used by the ruling Turkish "pashas".

After traveling for a couple of long days and nights, it felt good to get on our swimsuits and experience the hot mineral baths, a swim, and a shower—or two. We had to be quite the sight for these local Hungarians. This old bus full of foreigners, pulling suitcases out on the lawn to find those swimsuits.

Go-Teams was well organized; they had been hosting out-reaches for years. The bus carried close to 30 people including luggage, sleeping bags, and the majority of our food for the three-week journey. The only meat we had were large cans of corned beef. During that three-week trip we had corned beef spaghetti, corned beef tacos, corned beef everything. It was our main entree, and it wasn't bad, it was good, well, with a bunch of seasonings.

We were only in Budapest a day and soon back on the two-lane highway headed east to the Romanian border. We arrived at the border in the evening, and what a process we faced. The government was still in chaos after the recent execution of their dictator, Ceausescu and his wife. Westerners from multiple countries seeking entry into Romania were definitely suspect.

Bibles were considered contraband by the border guards. They did not want Bibles brought into the country. Of course, we had hundreds of Bibles stuffed in every available space including our personal luggage. The officer in charge gave the order to search—take us apart—and they did. We unloaded luggage from the compartments under the bus; they went through whatever they wanted. Little did this officer know that he was dealing with Sverker, whom I later named the Guard Whisperer. I believe he asked if we had Bibles, and the two men moved away from us, speaking in low voices for some time. Eventually the officer gave the order to stamp our passports and admit us into the country. I often wonder if that guard became a Christian after his encounter with us that evening. I am pretty sure Sverker slipped him a Bible.

Once through the border, we continued to drive in the early hours before dawn in hopes of getting to Bucharest within the next day or so. I was often Sverker's copilot and in charge of keeping him awake and alert. I would tell him stories of life in the country music business, firsthand interactions with the stars, musicians and staff and hanging out backstage at The Grand Ole Opry. I would tell stories of my childhood in the south, embellishing only where necessary. I loved Sarah Cannon and her alter ego, Minnie Pearl, at The Grand Ole Opry. I had told Miss Minnie, one evening backstage, that I could relate to her famous line, "I rarely let the facts interfere with the story." Whatever I needed to do to keep our driver awake, that's what I did... embellish, and exaggerate, but we kept laughing and driving.

One morning at a pit stop one of our team pulled me aside to tell me that she understood my job was to keep him awake, but she went on to say, "But not the entire bus." Hmmm, guess we did laugh a lot, and maybe a bit too loud.

Just before dawn that morning, we drove into a small city. There were people already moving about on the dark streets. We were already moving slowly, but suddenly, in an instant, Sverker braked hard, bringing our bus to an immediate halt. I asked him what was wrong, he said he had sensed danger and felt he should stop. Though we did not see anything in our path, in just a few seconds an old streetcar appeared out of the darkness and crossed directly in front of us. There were no lights on the streetcar, but if we had been a meter further, the streetcar would have broadsided our bus. God was again showing us that He was with us.

Once we had left the comforts of the west, there were almost no public toilets, and if there were, they were so unkempt that finding a tree was often a better option. Our first morning in Romania, we stopped where the cornfields were on each side of the road. Yep, girls on one side, boys on the other. You have 10 minutes!

Later that afternoon, we were heading east toward Bucharest when all of a sudden there was a loud bang, metal grinding bang, and the bus slowed and rolled to a stop on the side of the highway. Something was badly wrong. A couple of guys who had mechanical knowledge slid under the bus only to emerge with the report of a broken axle. Here we were on a highway in Romania, in an old Swedish bus with a major mechanical issue. Where were we planning to find a new axle?

Coming toward us on that two-lane highway was an old horse-drawn hay wagon driven by a man, his wife by his side, and two or three children in the back. Sverker grabbed my arm and said let's go and hitch a ride. He spoke to the family in German, I believe, and within seconds we were on the back of that hay wagon. The family was probably somewhere between shock and fear as they must have thought they had picked up Martians. We used our smiles to hopefully disarm them as we traveled up the road headed for the small Romanian city of Sibiu.

Once in Sibiu, we found our way into the center and found a taxi stand. Sverker, being Swedish, spoke at least a few languages, which was super helpful in negotiating. He found who appeared to be the ringleader of the taxis and paid for every taxi they could gather. He then jumped into one of those taxis, leaving me to lead the rest back to the bus.

There I stood in the middle of Sibiu, Romania, with no language skills, dressed in western attire, waiting on drivers with whom I would not be able to communicate. Try as I might, I was unable to blend in with my American tennis shoes and a smile, both of which were way too white.

Eventually the team and all of our belongings were transported into a very basic campground, somewhere in Sibiu. There were a number of large groups already camping when we arrived. Our group was the talk of the camp, and the town, I am sure.

Finding replacement parts for the axle took a couple of days and during that time our group set up camp, cooking the corned beef dishes, found local vegetables to purchase, and did our best to befriend these warm Romanian people. A few of us managed to invite ourselves into other camps and even joined in with some Romanian dances.

One of my favorite stories is about a soldier who was sent to *protect us*. He was most likely just doing his required year of service in the military. We were told that he was sent to protect us but he was probably sent to spy on us. We were extremely suspect. This young man stood nearby in his army uniform with his military-issued rifle across his chest. He had a menacing look on his face and stood there hour-after-hour, standing, watching, keeping us safe. It was hot, middle of the summer, and he was in a wool uniform complete with a gray green wool coat. My heart went out to him and occasionally I would look over and smile at him, and he would avert his eyes to avoid mine. This went on for a while. Some of our team were cooking in our large pots and the smells were wafting throughout the camp. When our dinner was ready, and we gathered to eat, I just thought how hungry he must be. At some point I decided I would make him a plate of food and take it to him. As I slowly strolled toward him I was determined to stay steady and just continue to smile and look him in the eyes. At first, he looked away, then back again, then away, like he did not know where to look... or what to do. Then he seemed to focus on the plate of food. He then would glance from the plate, to me, then back again to the plate. In a few more steps I was close enough to 'throw caution to the wind' and offer him the food. I could see now that he was only a boy, probably not more than 18-years-old. He put his gun down by his side, took the plate, and for the first time, he smiled. I have a picture of this young man eating and smiling while I am wearing his army hat and holding his rifle. It is one of my favorite photos not only because it evokes a good memory, but also it is a great reminder that I can't judge a book by its cover, or a person by the expression on their face. Sometimes we just have to reach out and take a chance!

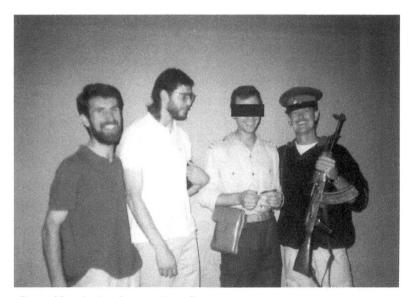

Daniel, Tim, Soldier, Randall, Sibiu, Romania 1990

Eventually the bus axle was repaired and our team was back on the road to Bucharest, the capital of Romania. Finding a campground on the edge of Bucharest, our group settled in for a week of street outreaches. We had a well-rehearsed mime drama called The Maze (the Labyrinth), Frontrunner would sing, and Sverker would deliver a Gospel message. We gathered large crowds anywhere we set up, whether on a square in downtown Bucharest or in the campground. People were hungry to hear our message, any message from *the west*. After praying for people we would give them Bibles and they would push in toward our team for those Bibles. Sometimes we were concerned that someone would be crushed.

After a week in Bucharest it was time to break camp and load up again for another road trip south to Bulgaria. Bulgaria, like Romania, is a beautiful country. We traveled there without incident, despite another long border crossing, but finally arrived in Sofia, the capital. What a beautiful old city. There were lots of what we would call Art Deco buildings in need of restoration, but the beauty still showed through. We set up in a campground just on the edge of the city and prepared for another week or so of out-reaches in downtown. As we did in Bucharest, we worked with the local churches. We hoped to encourage them as much as possible, as much as they would let us. These were early days of their *freedom*, and some of the pastors did not always trust westerners.

We witnessed incredible responses to our ministry outreaches. The communist system had failed people, and they were hungry, hungry for food, and hungry for truth. Food items were sparse so people had to borrow and barter. We were blessed to have our meals with us, even if corned beef was getting tiresome by that time. Sometimes after an outreach, some of us might go into a local restaurant to get some food, but more often than not the menu was extensive, but in reality, they might only have one or two items to prepare.

One morning, as we were leaving the campground heading into downtown Sofia, we received a message from one of the pastors. The old soviet office building was on fire. This was where we were planning to set up for our outreach. The fire was extin-guished quickly and we eventually had our ministry time a bit further down the promenade.

Leaving Bulgaria, beginning the long trip back to Amsterdam, we had to cross the Socialist Federal Republic of Yugoslavia from east to west. I will never forget my first glimpse of the Adriatic, glimmering as we approached that sea of aqua blue water. We drove into the seaside town of Opatija, (Croatia) and stopped the bus in front of the Hotel Belvedere. It was a beautiful hotel in its Austrian-Hungarian style, and it had recently been refurbished. Sverker decided that we needed a bit of reward for three weeks of campground showers, squatty toilets, and corned beef cuisine.

He went into the Belvedere and came back a few minutes later with the most amazing announcement. It seemed that there were unused outreach funds, and we were checking into the hotel for the rest of the day and night. At that moment we went from tired and weary travelers to the happiest bus of people on the planet.

Tim Berlin and I shared a room with a balcony looking out on that beautiful sea. After a shower I put on a clean white terry-cloth robe, provided by the Belvedere, but quickly found my swim trunks and down to the sea for a swim, then back again for another shower. Hot water!

That evening the team met for a nice dinner in the dining room. We swapped stories of the sea and the afternoon of warm showers and bathrobes. We were thankful to be clean and cool. We gave sincere thanks for so many amazing people we had met during our adventures over the past few weeks. What a precious gift in which to end a challenging but beautiful outreach.

21

Robbed At The Budapest Citadel

After the Summer of Service in Amsterdam, and outreaches in Eastern Europe, I decided to enroll in a Discipleship Training School (DTS) with YWAM. I had applied to the YWAM ship, Anastasis, and was accepted, but later learned that their proposed outreach was planned for West Africa. Though I loved West Africa, my heart was really aching to return to Eastern Europe. I had experienced so much in my visit to Berlin in '89 and during our recent outreach. I met with Maureen Menard who was leading the DTS department and asked if I could change my location to Amsterdam. Maureen met with her team; I was approved and accepted for the autumn DTS.

The lecture phase was in De Poort, where we gathered for lectures, slept, and ate our meals. Having been independent for a number of years, moving into dormitory-like accommodations was a bit of a challenge for me. I did have a private room, but it was in the area of the building that was badly in need of renovation. But I persevered, and at the end of the 12-week lecture phase, we boarded another old YWAM bus and once again crossed Europe.

Hal Young was our outreach leader from Atlanta. He drove the team from Holland to Hungary. Arriving in Budapest, we checked into the Citadel Hotel. The citadel (fortress) had been built in 1851 on Gellért Hill, high on the Buda side of the city. It remains a symbol of oppression as well as liberty. Sadly, in the Hungarian Revolution of 1956, Soviet troops occupied the Citadel and fired down into the city during the assault that overthrew the Nagy-led Hungarian government.

The hotel was in that old fortress built of stone walls a meter thick. It didn't take us long to figure out that something *dirty* was going on, as late at night on your trip down the hall to the bathrooms, you would often encounter scantily dressed women. One evening, on the way to the showers, I passed a door where two bodyguard-looking dudes stood outside with menacing looks on their faces. Obviously, the *godfather* was in that room working out his salvation *without fear and trembling*.

Our team was there to be a light in the darkness so we were not put off. However, the clincher came one morning when our team accountant went to get cash out of the hotel safe, but discovered our 14,000 Deutsche Marks—were gone! Yep, a hotel employee had made off with our cash, our team budget for the next three months. They left us lots of shredded paper, but no money to continue the outreach. Calls were made to YWAM Amsterdam; arrangements were made for replacement funds to be sent to us. Legal proceedings began with the hotel, who eventually, over time, paid the money back by hosting and housing YWAM teams for the next couple of years.

So our team moved and we spent Christmas of '90 at the Hotel Flandria on the Pest side of the city. During the days and some evenings our team worked with local churches doing music and dramas in the open squares of Budapest. We had tremendous response in those early days: there was real hunger for spiritual information.

In the weeks that led up to Christmas, one of our teammates, Winton Nicholson, came up with the idea of creating a trio to sing Christmas songs on the streets. He was a great singer, and multi-talented in dance and theatre in his home of Kona, Hawaii. Enock Freire, another team member, was from Brazil and also a talented singer and guitar player. The three of us harmonized well together. We rehearsed a few Christmas songs and soon decided to take our few songs to the streets.

We sang only Christmas songs at first, in the Metro station corridors just below the streets but before heading down to the Metro tracks. We also sang on the Váci Utca (Vaci street) one of the main pedestrian thoroughfares and perhaps the most famous street of central Budapest. Just off of the Váci Ut was the first Mc-Donald's fast food restaurant in Hungary. For our western team that was an oasis of *normal* and frequented often for those wanting a taste from home. Morgan and The Tramps would often sing on the streets near that McDonald's.

Those were hard days for the local people, so you rarely saw anyone smiling on the streets. When we started singing, the passersby would glance our way, and at times, we would get a slight smile, but people did not stop. After a few attempts at busking, Winton suggested that we place the guitar case in front of us, allowing people to tip. I was immediately uncomfortable with the idea as we were the rich people living in a hotel with three meals per day. This meant we were richer than most of the people in the city at that time. So I was against it, feeling embarrassed that we could even appear to be asking people for money. But Winton convinced me that it was worth a try. What a learning experience for me. Though they were only one cent forints and other coins not worth the metal on which they were printed, it changed the atmosphere and people began to stop. Some tipped, some did not, but having that opportunity made them feel safe to stop and listen to us. We began to draw crowds, which meant we needed to learn some more songs.

With Christmas over, it was time for our team to split again into two smaller teams: one to Romania and the other north to

Prague. I was on the Romanian team as assistant leader under Amsterdam staffer Dwayne Roberts.

The train from Budapest to Bucharest, Romania, was long and arduous. The conditions were not ideal. The old train bathrooms were not clean. The border crossing from Hungary to Romania, in the middle of the night, seemed to take forever. As the westerners on the train, we may have been the holdup. In great detail the guards went through our bags and studied our passports and our faces. Outside the train they shined lights under each carriage, checking for stowaways, even though the temperature must have been well below freezing. I remember arriving in Bucharest—and as cold and dark and desolate as it felt—it was good to be off of the train. Our small team split again in order to be housed with host families. That was a very hard winter for Romania. Food lines were long with literally only one or two items on the shelves of the stores. I remember one store only having bottled green beans. Bread was scarce and people awoke way before dawn to queue up for bread, a major staple in their diets.

Winton, Enoch and I stayed in a pastor's home in a high rise flat in downtown Bucharest. The three of us slept on a pullout sofa bed, which was really only large enough for two. The family were lovely and super hospitable to us, but it was a labor of love. There was little space for their family of four already, and now we were three more heads, mouths to feed, baths to be taken in the one small bathroom. We brought our own funds to pay for food and utilities, but finding food was a challenge. Moving into the new year of '91, we were appreciative for every bite we had during that hard, cold winter.

When we were not singing in orphanages, school assemblies, churches or ministering with the team, Winton, Enoch and I continued to practice, adding songs to our repertoire. We enjoyed sharing the gift of music with these wonderful people who had survived so much and had so little. This was my second time in Romania—though I did not know it at that time in the years to come I would be a regular visitor to this beautiful country.

After a few weeks in Romania, we returned to Budapest to rejoin the entire team. After some sharing about our times in Bucharest and Prague, we returned to Amsterdam for our final week of debriefing and graduation of our Discipleship Training School.

22

Morgan and The Tramps /

Marrakesh Express, Morocco

Spring of '91, after our DTS, our musical trio decided to literally *take it to the streets* by doing a 2-month European tour.

The three of us had been singing in Budapest as a street band. It was fun and well-received. Winton decided that we should be called Morgan and the Tramps. Though he sang most of the leads, I was the oldest. *Tramps* came from the thoughts of Corrie ten Boom's book, *Tramp for the Lord*. It did not have anything to do with *Lady and the Tramp* or any other less than desirable *tramp* terms. For us, singing/*tramping* was a fun way of meeting the people of a city. In Budapest we performed mainly in the underground chambers of the Metro stations, and on the Váci Utca. (Pedestrian street considered the heart of Budapest for shopping and restaurants.)

We hitchhiked from Amsterdam to Paris, from there on through Spain, to the Rock of Gibraltar. After a fitful night in sleeping bags under a dry-docked boat in Gibraltar, the next morning, we ferried from Spain to Tangier, Morocco. The ferry crosses The Straits of Gibraltar, a narrow strait that connects the Atlantic Ocean to the Mediterranean Sea, separating the Iberian Peninsula in Europe from North Africa.

Once in Tangier, we began working our way through the city in order to find the Marrakesh Express. Having been a Crosby,

Stills, Nash fan in my teens, taking the Moroccan train was almost surreal. It was on that overnight train that Graham Nash penned the words… "Wouldn't you know we're riding on the Marrakesh Express, they're taking me to Marrakesh".

After a day or so in Marrakesh we wanted to go deeper into the country so we took a public bus across the High Atlas Mountains to Quarzazate. There were more than a few moments when I was sure that old bus full of people, and a number of farm animals, would overturn, sending us down the side of the mountain. But we made it. Once safely in the ancient walled city, we were amazed at the beauty. The blue skies with billowing white clouds are some of the most beautiful that I have seen. Quarzazate and surrounding area is a noted filmmaking location, with Morocco's movie studios hosting many big name films. It is nicknamed *the door of the desert,* the gateway to the Sahara.

After a week of kicking around the old hippie trail of Morocco, we returned to Europe by ferry and hitched rides north to Ciudad Real, Spain. The Tramps resumed rehearsals, adding a number of new songs to our repertoire. After some rehearsal days, and time with friends, we headed back to Madrid, then on to Barcelona, singing and seeing some local sites in those beautiful cities. Then to Switzerland. We *worked* the streets of Geneva, Lausanne, Bern and Zurich, busking, making enough each day for food, and youth hostel beds, most evenings. We did not know that it was illegal to busk in some places, so we were taken to the Police Station in Milan, Italy. After a coffee we sang for the officers in the precinct and with smiles and handshakes they sent us back out to Tramp on. Singing in Venice and Rome was allowed, or so it seemed, because we were not arrested. We busked our way through Austria, a number of days in Vienna, before returning to Budapest. After some reunion time with friends we began our journey west, through numerous cities in Germany, back again to Amsterdam.

Those were some challenging months, but overall a great learning experience. Busking through Europe was a great way to meet people and share with them about the love of God.

After a few days back at De Poort, in Amsterdam, it was time to book flights home. Winton and Enoch would be returning to their homes in Kona, Hawaii, and I to Nashville. Before departing it was decided that I would apply for staff at the College of Performing Arts, YWAM's University of the Nations, in Kona, Hawaii.

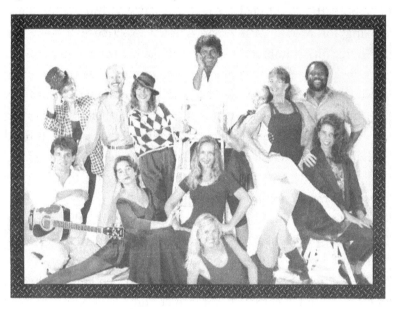

DOUBLE PORTION
THEATRE•DANCE COMPANY

Winton's mother, Gail Nicholson, was the Dean of the College of Performing Arts. Along with her friend and fellow dancer, Kate Waddle, they had developed the theatre troupe: *Double Portion.* Though I was only in Kona, autumn of '91 through spring of '92,

Gail and Kate were excellent leaders for me. Those were early years in my *Christian walk*, and I learned so much from them… their Grace-filled style.

In addition to lectures, dance and theatre training, I enjoyed teaching voice at the college. We were also busy rehearsing for Double Portion's California Tour, spring of '92. It included a show in the amazingly beautiful Avalon, on California's Santa Catalina Island.

Soon after that tour I learned that YWAM International was looking for people with organizational experience to plan the '92 Barcelona Summer Olympic outreach. I soon found myself back in Europe. The first month, in Barcelona, planning evening musical outreaches, near the Olympic Village. They ran from July 25–August 9. Being part of this team was another great learning experience. After the closing ceremonies, exhausted, I trained to Lausanne, Switzerland and crashed for a few days on David and Becky Durham's sofa… before continuing on to what was becoming my second home, Budapest, Hungary.

I was only in Europe a total of three months that summer. My father's health had been in decline and he wanted me to come home and I wanted to get a bit more time with him. I flew home in August and spent some time with him in September. Quietly, in his recliner, Dad crossed over into eternity one evening in early October, 1992.

— 23 —

Grieving What Could Have Been

In my late 30s a counselor said to me, regarding my relationship with my father, "You couldn't help from feeling belittled by your father when you were young, but you are an adult, and now you can help it." In my father's last years of life, I had to develop new responses to his negativity. When visiting him, it became my responsibility to redirect him, stop him, or go home. At first, I went home often, but I always phoned him, once I had arrived, just to say, "Dad, I am home. I don't want to talk now, just wanted you to know that I am safely home." I would tell him that I loved him, he would respond that he loved me, then I said goodbye and hung up the phone. I knew despite his harsh words that he would worry about me and would feel badly. I had to learn to parent my father.

I probably felt deep inside of my soul that I had let him down for just being me. I was a disappointment to him, and to myself, and for most of my younger years, I felt I was a disappointment to God. Even after my encounter with Jesus in '88 (going to Africa, moving to Africa as a missionary in '89), he still said, "I pray every day that you will come back to the church." He meant the Church of Christ. It was his opinion that the Church of Christ was *right*, and everyone else was *wrong*. My father could never shake the belief that it was about works and not by grace that one is saved.

I was in Dallas when my father passed. We had talked on the phone on my 40th birthday, just a day or two before. He said to me in that conversation, "I just hope that I have done enough." He was saying this with the fear he had lived with his entire life. He hoped the good he had done would outweigh the bad, and that he would go to heaven. I told him that it is *God's* grace that saves us... NOT our works. Jesus came to earth and died for our sins not to bring us a religion, but to bring us into relationship with Him. I knew that my father had that relationship, but he was still steeped in fear. I assured him Jesus died for us as His gift of salvation. It was truly that—a gift. I hope that my words brought him a bit of peace in his final hours.

A couple of days after that conversation with my father, his wife, Helen, called me in Texas to tell me that he had passed, slipped away quietly in his favorite chair. Helen married my father when they were both 65 years of age, and they were married for 10 years. She was a delightful woman, kind and hospitable. She was good to him and good to his sons.

I admit to having some degree of mixed emotions that evening when she called with the news of his passing. There was a part of me that felt peace knowing that my lifelong challenge of trying to gain his approval was over. I was free, on one hand, but on the other hand there was grief. I believe that sometimes we grieve not so much for what we had, but for what we should have, could have, had.

I am thankful for the Lord's healing in my life, which has included giving me much more grace for my father. He was tormented by many memories of his own past and childhood. When I think of him now, I remember the good times, and there were good times. I often wish that he were here today so that I could put my arms around him, give him a big hug, and tell him that I love him. Oh, how I look forward to the reunion on the other side; I know we will meet again.

After my father's funeral, I remained in Nashville for some months. I took a few interior design jobs over the winter. Spring of

'93 I enrolled in Grace Ministries Internship Counseling program to learn more about lay counseling and working with people who were struggling with all kinds of life challenges. I felt pretty experienced in dealing with life challenges.

The following summer I was back in Europe where I would staff a few Schools of Worship, organized by Musicians for Missions out of Amsterdam. They were hosted in Romania and Hungary, in '93 and '94. After the summer tour in '94, I made the decision to move to Budapest full time. Though I would travel, speaking and singing throughout the region, Budapest was my home for 7 years.

Spring of '95 I returned to Amsterdam for a few months to staff a MFM, School of Worship. At the end of the lecture phase, the students would travel to another country and minister in music for some weeks before returning to Amsterdam for the conclusion and debriefing of the school. It was during that school that I met David and Evelyne (Oprel) Lloyd. Dave was a great guitar player from Panama City, Florida and Ev played the flute and sang. So I recruited them along with singers Cathy Carter (Heiser) and Heather Loux (Myers) to resurrect Morgan and the Tramps. When the teams were sent out, we traveled to Budapest and joined the YWAM-Budapest-SOS (Summer of Service) with Hungarian youth, leading outreaches from Hungary to Bulgaria.

Morgan and the Tramps would continue to live on for many years. Dave and Ev became a main staple in the group until their family grew and then they helped train Tramps groups. Each year we would recruit young people to join us for street singing in Hungary, Romania, Bulgaria, Serbia, Bosnia, Croatia, Turkey, Poland, Slovakia, Czech Republic, and numerous countries in western Europe. Touching hearts with so many nations opened a door in my heart to create what would later become an international festival in southern Hungary.

RTL Klub 'Fókusz',
Hungarian Television

Dr. Petracek, my surgeon, and Dr. Mark Glazer, my cardiologist, at that time agreed that I should stay home, in the States, for at least one year after the surgery. For obvious reasons, they wanted to monitor my progress. But my home was in Eastern Europe. I had lived there for three years and the majority of what I owned was in my Budapest apartment. I wanted to go back. April of '98, six months after my surgery, I boarded a plane and returned to Hungary. What a great reunion! I had not seen most of these friends since I left in October under a cloud of doubt and fear. Now, here I was returning, with a new lease on life and blessed beyond belief.

When I landed in Budapest, good friends Steve and Barbara Johnson met me at the airport. It was an emotional meeting. It was at Steve and Barb's house just months before that we had prayed on that Monday evening after my diagnosis. Understanding the gravity of the situation, we prayed intensely for my healing. Steve had offered to stay with me at my apartment that night as he was concerned for me to be alone, and he drove me to the airport when I flew out on Wednesday morning. Steve was my last hug leaving Budapest and my first hug returning.

After delivering my luggage to my apartment in Zugló, we drove to the Hotel Góliát where the YWAM DTS International Collaborative was in full session.

Upon arrival, we slipped into the back of the large meeting room. Maureen Menard was teaching and saw me immediately, but continued her lecture. Then a few of the staff standing in the back started making their way toward me to give me a hug. Then others noticed and got up from their seats to come to me and finally Maureen just stopped. She laughingly said that she was going to introduce me at the break, but since she had lost the crowd.... . She was not upset, she understood. It was in those moments when I realized just how widespread the call for prayer for me and my situation had extended. These students were from a number of nations, and a good number had heard of my situation, and prayed for me in their YWAM Schools or in their churches. I was touched by the outpouring of love and the realization that so many had prayed. This was before social media platforms, yet the word traveled quickly across Europe and across continents within The Church, and YWAM networks. God heard their prayers and now they were expressing that to me in person.

Recently, Steve Ashworth, who lives in Amsterdam, reminded me that he had prayed for me while in Northern Iraq. Friends *down under* in Australia and New Zealand, in the Pacific Islands, The Americas, across Africa and Europe... the people of God were asking for my healing. That is extremely humbling and I am thankful for each person who prayed for me.

I had only been back a few weeks when the Hungarian television, RTL Klub show *Fókusz* (Hungarian equivalent to *20/20* or *60 Minutes)*—contacted me wanting to film a piece on my story. The Hungarians were extremely proud of the fact that their doctors had diagnosed my condition correctly. The Cardiology Hospital in Holland and the initial test in Nashville had not seen the dissection which could have cost me my life. A fact… that *Fókusz* pointed out in their feature piece. The vignette opened with me in my Budapest apartment, then did a nice interview with my cardiologist Dr. Mározsán. They showed translated clips of the Saint Thomas commercials, before ending with local video of me arriving at my flat on my bicycle, after cycling through the city— alive and well.

In a recent visit and conversation with my heart surgeon, Michael Petracek, he reminded me that had the Dutch hospital performed an echocardiogram, and had seen the dissection, they would have immediately scheduled emergency surgery, and my outcome, most likely, would be different. Europe, at that time, had organ banks, but not tissue banks. Therefore, my replacement materials would have been a mechanical or pig tissue valve and a synthetic Gore-tex® sleeve replacing the 4 inches of torn aorta. Dr. Petracek believes, as I do, that God had a plan, and despite all the drama, the misdiagnosis, exercise, even the prescription blood thinners—through it all God's plan was to get me home so that my surgery could have the best options for my recovery and longevity.

— 25 —

Cluj-Napoca, Romania to

Balástya, Hungary

Six months after my life-changing surgery I returned to Hungary and immediately began working on finalizing plans for that very summer. We were starting the festival in southern Hungary. Nine months almost to the day after my surgery we hosted the first Rock for Life festival.

For a number of years, some friends and I had been planning to create a Hungarian-based international festival. We had talked about it since attending the Cristea Festival in Cluj, Romania, in the early to mid 90's.

The year leading up to my heart episode we became more serious about finding a location and moving forward with an event that would bring people together from the region for the purpose of training leaders, especially in the area of the arts. We believed that these young bands and visual artists could become *agents of change* for their cultures in the quickly changing post-communist controlled Central and Eastern Europe.

The vision behind the festival began in a campground in Cluj-Napoca, Romania, in the summer of '93. Though the Cristea festival was beautiful on a number of levels, the most important was that young Christians wanted concerts and wanted more freedom than some of their traditional churches offered. Romanians love to sing and there were a number of bands and worship groups that attended the festival. There were also a few foreign bands, including our band from MFM in Holland and the YWAM Budapest musicians. Everyone attending camped, and that was great for the first day or so, before the campground manager decided that he could get more money, most likely for his own pockets, by raising the rent on the place. When the leadership refused, he cutoff the campground water. He claimed there was a problem due to the volume of people using the toilets, showers, etc., but in reality, he was the problem. In just a few hours the toilets were overflowing and there was very little water in the camp, so people were forced into the woods and forest around the campground, which wasn't good. In the end, I think some arrangement was made, a bribe most likely, and the water was restored. But not before making a huge and irreversible toilet problem.

It was during that week that we decided that we could create the festival in Hungary where there was a better infrastructure at that time. Because Hungary bordered Austria, it had seen more involvement with the West during the soviet-controlled years.

With my YWAM Budapest friends we decided that we could host an international festival in Hungary which was also more accessible to the neighboring nations. Hungary was bordered by seven countries (Slovakia, Ukraine, Romania, Serbia, Croatia, Slovenia and Austria). With additional three countries able to access Hungary without complicated travel visas. So we looked for a campground that could accommodate travelers from a number of nations, along with at least one hotel that could house an international team unable to camp.

Eastern Europeans were excellent at networking so we put the word out that we were looking for a camping facility in southern Hungary. Soon we heard of a family that worked with prostitutes and trafficking along the truck routes in that area. Yugoslavia's government fell in the '90s, and this family had to leave and move to southern Hungary, where they bought a farm on the highway from Budapest to Szeged, the southern city of Hungary near the Romanian and Serbian borders. Szeged is the 3rd largest city in Hungary.

The Davies family offered us their farm on that stretch of highway. We decided we would create our own little Woodstock, if you are old enough to remember the hippie festival in August of '69 in the United States.

Like Woodstock, Rock for Life would be a camping event, but we still needed housing for the international team and speakers who would be traveling in by air. A hotel would be important for a pre-team as well as a staff team for the festival itself. Balástya, Hungary, was a small spot in the road on that highway. It had one hotel that was pretty new and had an adequate number of rooms upstairs and a dining hall/event space on the main floor. It was also near the farm and though small, it would work. I knew that by doubling, tripling or quadrupling people in each room we could host the western teams from churches in Atlanta, Nashville, and a few other international cities. The dining hall was large enough for our breakfasts and a meeting point for the staff before the event started.

Hal and Brenda Young were members of Mount Paran Church in Atlanta at that time and had recruited a team to come the week before to build toilets and showers. Those outhouse toilets were so nice that any hillbilly from the mountains of Tennessee or Georgia would have envied us. We hired a local man to dig a well in the field and we ran PVC pipe into the shower shack. He also dug a huge pit and the team built that bank of toilets over that pit. When the festival was over, we just had a backhoe put the dirt back into the hole.

Because we were on the family farm, we were drawing electricity from the farmhouse, which was not adequate for our sound, lights and refrigerating units that provided some food and drink for our campers. So we had to go to a neighbor's farm and ask if we could purchase electricity from them, and because money talks, they agreed. I have no idea what we paid them, but it was a blessing for them and for us. We then had to go into Szeged and purchase enough electrical cord to reach from one farm across the fields to the other. It may be a small miracle that no one was electrocuted during the week, not even a grazing cow.

We had no trees. None. Zero. The circus-style tent that we borrowed from a Pentecostal Ministry in Budapest was in the middle of this field on hard ground with broken and bush hogged stalks of prior year's decaying crops. It was a high-pitched tent which did help in some ways to at least allow some of the heat to rise into the pitch. Suffice to say, it was one hot week. We also had a smaller tent that housed some semblance of a food court, doubling as a seminar room. It was a place that had picnic tables and a vendor who sold lard sandwiches and drinks. It did provide shelter from the sun, and one afternoon from the rain, which was welcomed to bring a bit of relief from the heat. The heavens opened up, the rain came down at a deafening rate, and some musicians from Eastern Europe started playing and worship took over that tent. There was singing, praising God, under the tent and a number of young people who danced in the rain just outside the tent. There were many good memories from our first Rock for Life, but that is certainly one I hear mentioned, even now, when I see friends who attended that event.

The founders of Youth With A Mission, Loren and Darlene Cunningham taught seminars under that food court tent. Darrow Miller, Director of Food for the Hungry, also came and spoke to our few hundred international festival registrants... challenging them to get involved in shaping their nations for the cause of Christ.

Why would internationally renowned speakers and musicians come to a ragtag event for a week of worship, seminars and concerts? It simply was the only multicultural gathering of Christians in Central and Eastern Europe at the time. The Church, interdenominationally seeking God together under one tent... was truly amazing. Those dedicated young people standing in the baking sun, worshipping together in a number of languages, was the Spirit of God. Every tribe and tongue worshipping together before the Throne.

In those early years of the festival, we witnessed travelers arriving by cars, buses, hitchhiking, and even walkers... crossing borders in order to get to us. Some would come with only a loaf of bread and possibly a summer sausage in their pack. They would travel miles in order to attend this first-of-its-kind-event. These young people were hungry for *the things of God,* and we were amazed at the attendance each year.

The evening music concerts were advertised as *free to the public,* which brought in guests from Szeged and nearby villages. The stage was part of a bus that was created by Stevan from Germany: RoadStage Europe. The bus sidewall was lowered, which created a small stage. The bus worked great for us, but remember we are in a field, not a well-prepared field for such an event. The field was mainly broken off crops that had dried over from the prior year that it lay fallow. Once the week was finished, and it was time to tear down and depart, we discovered that the bus had settled into the sandy ground. It wasn't easily extracted. We eventually got a tractor to come and pull the bus out of the deep grooves that it had made for itself.

We were not a rich ministry so everything that was used in that first festival was repurposed, even the woodshed toilets and showers. All the wood was stored there on the Davies farm, and the following year, once we moved to an actual campground, we created a stage from that wood. It is amusingly notable that for years to come so many people asked why there were "Men" and "Women" stickers at various places on the SOZO Festival stage. That stage had seen a lot!

We were not there to just sing or be entertained or even to be taught about our walks with God by notables like the Cunninghams. We were there to celebrate what God was doing in each of our countries. We called out each nation in attendance and prayed for that nation. We prayed for these amazingly beautiful young people who had possibly spent all to get there. They had crossed many borders. They had walked and hitchhiked with determination to experience God in a festival atmosphere. I had traveled extensively through Eastern Europe over the past seven years, and I had worshipped in some of the churches from which they came. Churches where the men sat on one side and women on the other. The women wore head coverings—a hat or scarf. A number of their pastors had survived hardships through the years of communism, often persecuted, even imprisoned at times. They made less money than their peers, being denied privileges that the government doled out at its discretion. We encouraged them to honor these faithful pastors when they returned home.

We knew that these young people were going to experience freedom in worship that would give them thirst for more. After a week at the festival they would return to their home churches and struggle with the lack of *spiritual vitality* that they experienced at the festival. They had found freedom, whether simply clapping along with the modern worship choruses, raising their hands in surrender to God, or even dancing. But we were modeling something that would either change the existing churches of Eastern Europe, help to birth new churches, or both.

Birthing The International SOZO Festival

With the success of our first festival in Balástya, Hungary, we knew we would grow, and grow quickly in the years to come. We would need more developed space than the farm would allow. We needed an actual campground, with showers, toilets, and a stage area, nearby shops, restaurants, hostels and hotels. After a few weeks of rest from Rock For Life '98, this became my focus for the remainder of that year.

Soon I heard from a friend that there was a nice campground in Baja, Hungary, only an hour east of Szeged. So Hal Young, Steve Johnson, David Lloyd and I made a day trip to Baja, just two hours south of Budapest. We toured the campground and the little city, located where the Danube and Sugovica Rivers merge, just across from one of the largest protected forests in Europe, the Gemenc.

It had a lovely campground in the city center on Petőfi-sziget, what the Hungarians called their Sports Island. Sugovica Hotel and Kemping. That's right... *kemping*... not a misspelling. It is *kemping* in Hungarian. So the Sugovica Hotel and Kemping were exactly what we needed. The kemping area had wooden bungalows with small porches and plenty of space for tents. There was also a small cook house for campers and a brick shower house with nice sinks and toilets. In addition, just a short walk away, there was also a large field where there had been some sort of outdoor movie theatre. It was a raised area with a wooden plank outside floor and a large metal grid behind it. It was a great foundation for a concert stage!

We met the manager of the hotel facility, Angeli Mónika, and immediately liked her. I had no idea that day that I would work with her for many years to come and I am thankful that we continue to be friends to this day. Mónika was, and is, one of the nicest, most agreeable and professional people that I have ever worked with. She always did her best to accommodate this massive group of internationals.

Less than an hour from the Serbian and Croatian borders, two hours from Romania, Baja seemed perfect for an international event. We learned from some locals that it had been a city of reconciliation during the Yugoslavian war. Pastors on both sides of the border gathered there to pray for their former Yugoslavian home. It was a city of reconciliation! Wow! We felt that was where the Lord had led us for such a time as this. We had started out as a Music and Arts event but soon evolved into a festival focused on reconciliation and unity... unity among the nations, and denominations. Baja just felt right. It felt like a potential home for the festival.

Due to my travel throughout the region, I wanted the festival to be about bringing the nations together. When traveling through Eastern Europe and the Balkans, I would often hear the same comments in each country. They would ask, "Where have you come from?" I would reply the neighboring country; they would often respond, "Oh, you need to be careful." They warned of high crime, deception, danger by *those people*. But the lies were always the same. They had been taught lies about their neighbors, and, of course, they had believed them. The government controlled the news, and the propaganda machine was alive, and *not well* in Eastern Europe. I wanted to bring people together so that they could see how they were alike, as well as how they were different. At each event, our goal was to celebrate the beauty of their cultures, and to identify and applaud what God was doing in them individually and in their particular nations.

Our first festival in Baja, as with any new event, had its challenges: electrical, lighting and sound, food vendors, city officials who sought to make a bit of cash on the side. One evening we faced a problem with the city. Steve Johnson and I went to city hall on Szentháromság (Holy Trinity) Square. It was closed except for a security guard; he kindly telephoned Dancsa Bálint, the vice mayor of cultural events. Bálint lived nearby, and walked over that evening to meet with Steve and me. He quickly solved our problem and through the years became our advocate and a good friend.

After the first Rock For Life in Baja (summer of '99), I decided that a new name would be necessary. I was hearing reports that pastors in the region would not let their youth attend a *Rock Festival*. I tried to explain that the name was based on Jesus being *The Rock* of our Salvation but getting that word out was not so easy in the days before social media.

The festival needed a name change so I began the search. I wanted something simple that would not translate badly in one of the many languages in our ministry region. One might be surprised at how many little four to five-letter words mean something completely different in Slavic, Latin, and Hungarian-based languages.

During the winter of '99, I was home in Nashville for followup heart exams, fundraising, and to recruit teams for the coming summer. Mike Demus, a Nashville studio owner and producer asked, "Have you heard of the word sozo?" Sozo is a Greek word that means Healing, Salvation and Deliverance. What a great word with a great meaning, an actual proclamation or even a prayer for Eastern Europe. Just seemed like one of those God moments!

So the name was changed and the SOZO Festival was born, summer of 2000, in Baja. We had some amazing times of worship—multicultural and multilingual—every tribe and tongue worshipping before the throne of God.

There were times when the Spirit of God was so strong that you could feel his presence. I remember one morning during our worship, I was standing just inside the tent with tears rolling down my face. I was in awe of hearing these familiar songs being sung by hundreds of people from dozens of countries, same song, same meaning, but different languages. I was also reminded of how God had been so gracious to sustain my life, to add to my days. As I stood there basking in His presence, one of the staff came and whispered in my ear that we had a bit of a problem. That was not an uncommon thing to hear. As I walked out of the tent my tears immediately stopped and I went into work mode. If memory serves me correctly, the issue was simple, and I soon returned to the tent. Immediately as I walked back under the flap of the large circus tent, my tears began to flow again. The hair on the back of my neck stood up with a chill. I knew I was in the presence of something far greater and more majestic than I had previously experienced. I was in the presence of God. His people were singing praises to Him in multiple languages, and it was incredible. I will always remember that moment and the many God moments at SOZO.

One of the earlier years, we had a lone traveler from Croatia who had appeared at our gate. He had traveled for a few days to get to Baja, and had come on every possible mode of transport, including hitchhiking. He arrived with only a rucksack, and the small remains of a loaf of bread. The word went out through the camp that we needed a tent and a sleeping roll for this Croatian young man. Despite the war and the controversial NATO bombings in that area, it was the Serbs and Bosnian campers who graciously welcomed him into their camp. Late in the evening after this young Croat's arrival, I received a call on my walkie talkie that I needed to come to the campground. That was usually not a good call at night. I figured there must be a problem bigger than our volunteer security team was willing or able to handle. I got on my bike and pedaled as quickly as I could to where the majority of the participants were camping. As I dismounted my bike, all seemed peaceful with the night sounds of nature and people talking, singing, playing guitars around their campfires. As I moved toward the area of concern, I realized it was not a concern at all. I experienced something beautiful. The Serbs and Bosnians were worshipping with this Croatian young man. This group of former 'Yugoslavians' were worshipping God together singing in the *forbidden language* of Serbo-Croat. I still feel emotional telling this story. Those God stories of unity, forgiveness, and reconciliation became a banner of the SOZO Festival.

In 2015, after a few years of events in other countries, we returned to Baja. With Russia and Ukraine at odds over Crimea, it made it impossible for our Russian friends to travel to Hungary through Ukraine. Andrei, Lena and their daughters had been part of the festival for many years, not only in Hungary but also in Novi Sad, Serbia, and the UK. Being an important part of the SOZO family, they were determined to attend. They had to drive through Belarus, Poland, and Slovakia before entering Hungary. When they arrived, I watched Andrei get out of the car and look across the field to where our brother and staff leader, Karlos Horvath, was helping setup. Karlos is ethnically Russian Hungarian-Roma (Gypsy), raised in Munkachevo, Ukraine. Those men locked eyes, and with broad smiles, they sprinted across the field to each other locking into an embrace that could be paralleled to the father and son in the prodigal son story in the Bible. Brothers! Family! Despite the disagreements of their countries, the politics, the media and propaganda, the hearts of these friends were well above wars and rumors of wars. Brothers in Christ, with true affection for each other and their families.

These were just a few stories, among dozens if not hundreds of amazing God moments at the SOZO Festival. During our 18 years, the large majority of the festivals were in Hungary but with additional conferences in Romania, Serbia and the United Kingdom. Summer of '99 we partnered with missionary friends to host Rock For Life, Turkey, August of '99. Sadly, we arrived the day of a massive earthquake which killed over 17,000 people, injuring at least 45,000, and leaving more than 250,000 homeless. We were set up near the ancient Ephesus ruins, in Selcuk, but we could hardly have a festival when so many were hurting. We quickly redirected our efforts, taking our musicians into hotels and a few open air concerts to raise funds for the devastation of the 1999 Izmit Turkey earthquake.

Despite all of the different locations and the hundreds of staff and thousands of participants in these different countries, Baja, in southern Hungary, was our SOZO Festival home. It was our *special* place where God brought Healing, Salvation and Deliverance.

— 27 —

Hope That The Homograft
Will Last 15-20 Years.

In early November of 1997, in a followup post-surgery visit, my surgeon, Michael Petracek, told me that he "hoped" this aortic valve and sleeve, my homograph, would last 15 to 20 years. Recently, during my yearly checkup, Dr. Tom McRae was happy to report that "my" valve is still functioning correctly and we both agreed that it is truly a miracle. 2022 is my 25th year of living a very active life, with a human tissue valve and aortic sleeve. Someone kindly donated their organs and tissue to be harvested and stored for a person in need. That person in this situation was me and I am so thankful for that donor and hope one day on the other side in eternity that I may get to meet them and thank them.

Over the past 25 years I have had multiple doctors, nurses, interns, and students listen to my heart. Sometimes in their medical training and experience they simply have not heard a human donor valve. In addition to doctors and health care professionals in the USA and Hungary, I have been examined in the UK, Romania, Serbia, Croatia, and Brazil. I have had multiple echocardiograms, stress tests, and MRIs, to check my aorta from heart to stomach. I have been blessed with doctors who care for me and have taken true interest in my story, recovery and my future. I have in turn tried hard to do my best with diet and exercise. Living in different countries has, at times, made it difficult to follow a heart healthy diet. I have tried to stay active and fight against the high fat foods which I find to be delicious. Chicken paprikás, Hungarian töltött káposzta, Romanian sarmale, cevapi in Bosnia, Croatia and Serbia, schnitzels, fish & chips, steak & Guinness pie, bangers and mash, Yorkshire Pudding, not to mention England's Sticky Toffee Pudding... just to name a few.

In the writing of this book, I have been reminded again and again of the Lord's faithfulness to me. Coming from a challenging early home life, and the sadness of feeling alone, living under the cloud of that horrible whispered 'cancer' word, the sadness and fear, the self-doubt that my father lived with, the Lord has brought so much healing and has allowed me to experience a very full life.

Though my aortic dissection could have ended my life, or greatly reduced my ability to *go and do...* it has not. It did not stop me from an active missions and ministry career. It did not prevent me from joining with my friends to start the SOZO Festival... and lead 18 years of events. It did not prevent the hosting of multiple leaders from the U.S. and many nations at the SOZO House on Petőfi Sziget, in Baja, Hungary... a house provided by good friend and brother, Johan Blom, in the Netherlands.

It did not stop me from speaking, singing, ministering in over 50 countries. I am so thankful for all of these experiences and opportunities. One recent trip was at a large multinational Latino conference in Itajaí, Brazil. There were over 12 Latino nations represented. I experienced such warmth and love among these people. In speaking, I tried to encourage them in their local and global callings. The warmth and genuine affection displayed among the Latin people was amazing. That week was another reminder of how blessed my mission and ministry life have been.

As I look back, I am truly amazed of what God has allowed me to do.

My beginning years were self-absorbed in many ways. I want my next years to be all about people, helping people find hope and purpose in the way God has shown me hope and given me purpose.

28

Captain Morgan

After the 2006 festival I returned home to Nashville for a year before moving to the UK. Serving with a network of churches, speaking, training leaders in worship and outreach, I continued to travel within and out of the UK until the end of 2015, when I started to feel my international life in missions was coming to an end. Not an end to missions, and not an end to international missions, but an end to possibly living overseas on a permanent basis.

Moving back to my native Nashville was a hard decision for a number of reasons. My life and career had been in Europe for so many years. I have many friends and a large international family spread across the nations. I felt real purpose in ministry... that I would miss. But another factor was that I had bought a place to live in England. After many years of renting apartments from Nigeria, Hungary, Holland, Switzerland, to the midlands of England, I had purchased a *home*, a tiny house on the water, a canal boat. Long boat. A barge.

UK apartment rentals were expensive, and not so cozy. I found most apartments had paper thins walls and you could almost set your watch by your neighbors' activities. I began to think of alternatives and soon began a search for an old canal boat in need of renovation. I would target areas of the canals where boats were moored and walk along the footpath and visit with the owners. One afternoon, I met a couple who told me about two men that purchased boats on consignment, renovating them for resale. They recommended them to be honest and their work to be quality so I did some searching and found them in Tamworth, Staffordshire. The day I drove on to their lot they were working on an old barge named "Ben." It was being primed to paint, but the interior was dark and old, in my opinion, in bad need of gutting. After some days and a couple of visits, we came to an agreement with the marina owners, and the family who owned "Ben." Within a couple of months it had been completely renovated into my home. There is superstition around boats and water, and one of those was a boat should never be renamed, unless it had been taken out of the water. During the painting and hull inspection my newly purchased barge had been in dry dock so I was free to bless her with a new name. My mother's maiden name was Brown, and my parents passed it on to me as my middle name. I had often heard that the English think hyphenated names are *posh* so I decided that my newly renovated boat would certainly need to be posh, so I christened her the Morgan-Brown.

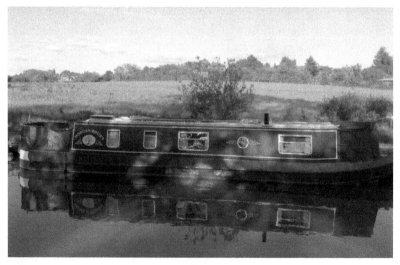

The Morgan-Brown Canal Barge, Midlands of England 2015

I was working with a group of churches in the UK, so I wasn't out cruising on a daily basis, but I did get a few local trips to the locks near Rugby where I rented a permanent mooring.

A bit over a year later, I made the decision to move back to the States. John Lee, a friend who owned Aspley Wharf Marina in Huddersfield, kindly offered to sell the Morgan-Brown for me. I would need to get it to Huddersfield. No problem, I thought, that is just a bit over 2 hours, 110 miles north on the M1... by car.

Despite my lack of confidence with anything mechanical, especially that diesel engine, I made the decision to make the voyage north to Huddersfield. I really had no idea, when I set out, what the daily maintenance would require. After each full day of travel, I had to remove a section of the deck and climb down into the engine. I learned to check fluids, grease the prop and clean out the prop box... anything foreign like leaves, trash, or possibly small critters that could have been floating in the canal. Yuck.

I did my research on the trip, routing through 138 miles of canals from North Oxford, Coventry, Trent and Mercy, Macclesfield, Huddersfield Canal into Yorkshire. With a few delays, mechanical and weather, it took me 18 days to arrive at my destination.

While researching I somehow missed the fact that I would need to travel through a couple of long tunnels along the way. I am claustrophobic! Possibly the result (PTSD) from almost drowning in Holland when my aorta dissected. When I set out for a three-week trip north, I was aware that I would hand crank myself through 144 locks, a couple of drawbridges—where I actually had to stop traffic before raising the bridge—and a number of small tunnels under roadways and the like. I did not know that I would have to brave the Hardcastle Tunnel on the Trent and Mersey Canal in Staffordshire, about an hour completely alone! Inside the tunnel was pitch black with nothing but the headlamp on my boat, an LED-lighted hardhat and an airhorn in my hand that would call for help, should I get stranded. The officer at the tunnel gate told me to blow the horn and *if* they heard it, they would send a boat in to help. If they did not, after more than an hour they would send a boat in anyway. Comforting.

But the most daunting challenge was when I arrived at the notorious Standedge Tunnel. A hand-dug tunnel, 3.5 miles (5,029 meters, 16,499 feet) long and only wide enough for one boat inside at a time. Its construction, beginning in 1790 was no easy feat - it took several engineers and 17 years to complete. The tunnel lies 636 feet, 194 meters beneath the stunning Standedge moors in the Yorkshire Pennines.

Thankfully, they send a guide in with every boat to keep an eye on the carbon monoxide levels and is knowledgeable of the location of the occasional cross tunnels… should you need to evacuate. I was also joined by my friend Gordon Williamson who was in charge of prayer, for the boat, and for me!

The Canal & River Trust calls it one of the seven wonders of the waterways! After surviving this one *wonder*, I don't really want to travel through the other six. My Canal & River Trust Certificate of Accomplishment, states *The Morgan-Brown has braved the darkness of the Standedge Tunnel.* I am very glad it does not mention the apprehensive Captain Morgan.

I did conquer some fears on that three-week trip. I often recited the 23rd Psalm. His rod and staff did comfort me, and though I was not walking, I was driving my boat-home through what seemed like the "valley of the shadow of death", He was with me. God "prepared a table before me in the presence of my enemies", which in this case were a diesel engine and my lack of mechanical abilities. Through it all, He was with me, I could feel His presence. I must say that living on the Morgan-Brown and that three-week trip remain a highlight in my years abroad.

29

Relationship Not Religion

L ike everyone else, my journey through life has had its ups and downs. There are always challenges. My childhood started in less-than-ideal circumstances that were hard for me, hard for my brothers, and hard for my parents. Yet, it probably looked ideal compared to some people's beginnings. I had a father and mother in the home, and I was loved, despite the lack of affection or the warm relationships that I desired. We did not get everything we asked for, yet we never went without.

Growing up in the Church, I wanted to know God. Yet He seemed so distant and truly knowing Him felt unobtainable. A relationship with the God of the universe was just impossible in my mind. We often get our picture of God from our earthly fathers. The lack of bonding with my *earthly father* most likely blocked me from knowing my *Heavenly Father*.

In '88 when I surrendered my life to Jesus, I understood for the first time that this was a relationship, not a religion.

Back in '89, I told some friends that I was thinking about leaving my Music Row career. When I told them of my plans to move to West Africa, one of them said to me, "Now wait, I know you have had a religious experience, but you're going to be okay ." meaning, you will get back to *normal*. I wanted all of God that I could have. Simply said, I did not want to be *okay* . I had not had a religious experience. I had an encounter with Almighty God. I wanted to live in His fullness.

I am amazed at what the Lord has allowed me to experience. Maybe you have heard it said that God does not call the equipped, He equips the called... and He certainly did that for me. Did He call me into missions over 30 years ago? I believe it was a calling, not an audible voice, but a desire to serve and bring hope to the hopeless. Did he provide all that I needed exactly when I needed it? He did. I have said many times that God is never late and I hope you will not think this is sacrilegious, but He does, however, miss a lot of chances to be early.

I am a broken vessel that spent the first half of my life wandering, searching for hope. In this second half, my desire is to help others find hope, peace and joy in their lives. I have learned to trust the Lord and do my best to follow the teachings of Jesus. Not to lean on my own understanding but trust Him in all of His ways.

My friend, author and TV host, Sheila Walsh, wrote, "My brokenness is a better bridge for people than my pretend wholeness ever was." I feel that is true for me as well. I now know myself well enough to be a bridge to help others find healing and hope.

When people tell me the reasons that they do not believe or are not interested in Christianity, I understand. I have been there. It is rare that someone tells me an opinion that I have not previously held.

If you are one of those people who cannot, will not, buy in to religion, I understand. But I ask you, please do not throw out the baby with the bathwater. God is alive, and His Son Jesus died for you. He came so that we might have a more abundant life. After His resurrection and ascension into heaven, He sent us the Holy Spirit. The Spirit is my comforter, He is my guide in life. He guided my steps from the lake in Holland to Budapest to Nashville. He ordained that I should live and not die to declare his Glory. *Psalm 118:17*

I hope you have understood that this is the message of my book. It is not about me, it is about Him. God the Father! He was never afraid of my doubts, my questions, and He is not afraid of yours. He pursued me, He waited patiently for me.

Those who know me know for sure that I have not reached any form of perfection but in the words of the Apostle Paul, and a beautiful hymn that I grew up singing, "… for I know whom I have believed, and am persuaded that He is able to keep that which I have committed unto him against that day." 2 Timothy 1:12

My hope and my prayer in writing this book is that you will give God a chance. He is not afraid of your questions, your doubts, your fears, your unbelief. Ask Him to reveal himself to you and I know that He will… just as He did for me. It was not my feeble attempt at prayer that Bloody Mary Morning in 1988, it was my surrendering to Him. He had been waiting, knocking on my heart's door. He stands at your door and knocks. *Revelation 3:20*

Acknowledgments

I would like to thank so many people who have invested in my life, but there is simply not enough space here. I do want to thank the following. Without you, this book may never have become a reality.

Erin and Peter Keene for your hospitality and generous encouragement.

Barbara Foster for your attention to detail and ability to banter.

Dave Flowers, Ranjeet Guptara, Austin Hardcastle, and Robbie Stofel for your input and encouragement to keep moving forward.

My international SOZO Festival Family from over 50 nations.

Cul2vate Monday morning church.

FRIENDS / Love Local, Community Church of Hendersonville.

CPSIA information can be obtained
at www.ICGtesting.com
Printed in the USA
BVHW052238221222
654897BV00012B/256

9 798987 112618